At The Center: A Place of HOPE, w(
Hannah lead training on very comple
ple and practical. I have read every p
she has succeeded again with fresh and practical applications in this
emerging area of mental health and neuroscience.

—Gregory L. Jantz, PhD, CEDS
Founder, The Center: A Place of HOPE

We have all struggled with the impact of living in a broken world,
some more than others. The impact of deep inner wounds can fol-
low an individual through a lifetime. Though in the past, inner
wounds can continue their damage in the present and threaten to
direct one's future. *Lasting Change* is a tremendous book for anyone
who longs for help to fight the powerful influence of the wounds of
the past. Hannah has written this gem to make the complexity of
the human mind understandable, giving the reader a roadmap of
practical application for freedom and real change.

—Tom Mulhern, MA, LMHC

Finally, a book that makes neuroscience of the brain easy to understand, plus enjoyable to read! At the end of each chapter are practical exercises. These can be used to explore and implement healthy,
long-lasting changes. Excellent book as a resource for therapists or
your average Joe looking for self-help!

—Michelle Morris, MSW, LISW-S
Owner of Open Gate Counseling and Consulting Services

LASTING CHANGE

Overcoming the Grip of Anxiety, Depression, & Trauma with "User-friendly" Neuroscience

LASTING CHANGE

Overcoming the Grip of Anxiety,
Depression, & Trauma with
"User-friendly" Neuroscience

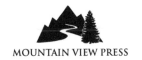

MOUNTAIN VIEW PRESS

HANNAH SMITH

Artwork created by Beth Eckel: www.doctorsartgallery.com

This book is not meant to provide medical advice nor to be considered a replacement for individual therapy with a professional.

Published by Mountain View Press, an imprint of Redemption Press, PO Box 427, Enumclaw, WA 98022.

Toll-Free (844) 2REDEEM (273-3336)

Redemption Press is honored to present this title in partnership with the author. The views expressed or implied in this work are those of the author. Redemption Press provides our imprint seal representing design excellence, creative content, and high-quality production.

Unless otherwise indicated, all Scripture quotations are taken from the Holy Bible, New International Version®, NIV® Copyright ©1973, 1978, 1984, 2011 by Biblica, Inc.® Used by permission. All rights reserved worldwide.

ISBN: 978-1-64645-132-6 (Paperback)
978-1-64645-133-3 (ePub)
978-1-64645-134-0 (Mobi)

Library of Congress Catalog Card Number: 2020907737

For the God who makes all things beautiful in their time;
my family, who let me run around the country teaching
and sharing my passion; and all the mighty and brave people
I have met along my journey:

Nothing is for nothing.

CONTENTS

AUTHOR'S NOTE

FOR SOME TIME now, I have been afforded the amazing privilege of sharing cutting-edge neuroscience information related to the treatment of anxiety-based mental health disorders with therapists all around the country. This has been a special honor for me. Not only am I a trained therapist and teacher with over twenty-five years of experience in clinical, educational, church-based, and even corporate settings, I am also a person with a "rewired brain."

As a survivor of chronic childhood trauma and diagnosed with post-traumatic stress disorder (PTSD) and dissociative disorders in my twenties, I experienced firsthand the tremendous shame and confusion inherent to such a life. My faith, along with learning the difference between biology and character, allowed me to see how truly wonderfully we are wired. These were the catalysts through which I learned to own my story. Slowly I have emerged from the pits of shame and have incorporated life experience, along with years of study, into my clinical practice. I have witnessed the shame-breaking benefits of understanding neuroscience innumerable times in my work. My hope now is that including this information in a book will help countless others.

There is much to say about this topic. However, most of the time, I train in brief, one-day sessions. Although the response has been overwhelmingly positive, it is quite clear it is next to impossible to learn and retain all the information shared in the training setting alone. This has resulted in multiple requests for a reference to capture not only what was taught in the seminar, but to also include the straightforward and uncomplicated manner in which it was conveyed. This book is the response to those requests.

Therefore, I have attempted to write this in the same engaging way I usually communicate it in a training session, with the hope of making it interesting, accessible, and appealing to survivors and healers alike. For those familiar with my presentation, the titles of various sections and chapters correlate to the seminar for easy reference. For use as learning tools, exercises, vignettes, and case studies are also included.

Please understand, this is a primer of sorts, not an exhaustive text. It is also not meant to be anatomically or scientifically precise at all times. The focus is on feet-to-the-ground understanding and implementation of complicated information. I direct my writing to you, the reader, and I address you as "you" and me as "I/me" rather than from a removed, technical, third-person perspective. Just as some movies are based on a true story, this is based on true science. However, it is also personal and should be taken as such. I try to exhibit the confidence I feel about this material in my writing, but if you feel the proverbial shoe does not fit in a particular instance, feel free to chuck it out!

Thank you for joining me as important principles for rewiring the anxious, depressed, and/or traumatized brain are shared and explained. The hard news: anxiety-based diagnoses are on the rise—exponentially so, it seems, these days. The good news: an understanding of the brain-body connection and a whole-person approach can provide significant relief to millions who struggle. Remember: go slow, breathe, ponder, and enjoy.

Let's begin.

PART I

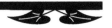

Foundations

CHAPTER ONE

Why Neuroscience?

What Difference Does the Brain Make?

I AM A SURVIVOR, but I wasn't always.

This may seem a funny way to open a book related to brain science and the treatment of anxiety. However, to make sense of the world in which we live, humans need context and story. We also need to be interested.

Currently, I work as a therapist and teacher—also known as a psycho-educator. However, my work history includes experience in clinical, educational, and even corporate settings—in both the US and India! On a more personal level, I grew up with a bipolar mother, a traumatized and angry father, and many experiences resulting in years of immobilizing fear, poor relationships, baffling self-destructive behaviors, and diagnoses of PTSD and other dissociative disorders.

Why do I tell you this? Because, I get it . . . and I am not alone. Millions of people in the United States (and around the world) struggle with anxiety-based mental health conditions, such as generalized anxiety disorder (GAD), obsessive-compulsive disorder

(OCD), social and other phobias, depression, and trauma. These conditions often greatly interfere with their daily lives.

According to the National Alliance on Mental Illness (NAMI), anxiety is the most common mental health disorder diagnosed in America (NAMI.org). Statistically speaking, in fact, you likely battle anxiety yourself, know someone who does, or treat it in others. Either way, you want to understand and conquer this beast. The hope is this volume will motivate you to learn some of the secret weapons you can use to defeat anxiety. Once you do, you will be likewise armed against many other common mental health disorders.

To begin, think about your own life story. Yes, you. Therapist or survivor, we all have a life story. What have been the obstacles on the path to wellness for you or for those with whom you work? Surely there have been many hurdles, but almost certainly one of them has been shame. Shame underlies nearly every mental health disorder and undermines all modalities of treatment. It can be thought of as an infection of the emotional system, which can leave a person feeling overwhelmed, defeated, and hopeless.

Many factors contribute to shame. Traumatic experiences, especially at the hands of powerful significant others in our lives, can be internalized as shame. Poor modeling may also result in a distorted sense of self and the world. Even being misinformed or misunderstanding people contributes to a negative self-image. Mental illness is mostly invisible and difficult to relate to by those who have not experienced it. Unhelpful platitudes ("Just get over it") and lack of self-understanding (not knowing why we do what we do) may leave us reeling and can chip away at our sense of self-worth.

Thankfully, modern neuroscience provides insight affirming what many of us have known about ourselves on some level all along—mental health issues are *not character flaws!* Understanding this provides a much-needed divide between what is disorder and what is not. Insight into how wonderfully we all are wired can help us see ourselves in a more accurate light and allow us to effect positive and lasting change.

As said above, I am a survivor *now*. There was a time, however, when I didn't know I was more than my brain and emotions. This kept me trapped and limited my options in life. For many years, I lived as a slave to a discordant array of bodily sensations and unsettling mental images. Seeking relief from these dictated my actions and shaped my core beliefs in dangerous ways at times. Through it all, I was convinced I had no choice but to do what I did. "It's just how I am" was the age-old saying I knew all too well and spouted regularly. Understanding neurobiology gave me the gift of my mind. Separating mind and brain allowed me to look at my life, my beliefs, and my actions in an entirely new and empowering way.

As for the question "What difference does the brain make?" the answer for me, and I hope for you too, is "All the difference in the world."

Okay . . . Tell Me More

Gladly. I will begin with some startling, earth-shattering, life-changing, watch-out-world news for you. Ready for it? Here goes: You are *not* your brain.

I can hear you now. "Huh? Wait a minute! You just told me in the last section the brain makes all the difference in the world!"

Yes. Yes, it does. Well, the knowledge of what it is does. The benefit comes from the understanding that we are more—immeasurably more—than our brains. Our brains are phenomenal and amazing, with a myriad of intricate functions. However, for our work as therapists or as those in therapy, it can be helpful to categorize brain functions as either conscious or nonconscious. Not everything we do is done with awareness. In fact, we spend an awful lot of time running on automatic.

With respect to running on automatic, it can be helpful to think of the brain as a simple binary, rule-based machine with two primary goals: safety and efficiency. When not mindful, the brain will make decisions and push us toward actions in keeping with these two goals.

An overarching function of the brain is to learn. This can happen as a more secondary process in the nonconscious, and as adults, we often prefer this. Learning, interestingly, may be the opposite of safety when done consciously. Think about it. Learning upends the process of efficiency and can be jarring. It can take time to develop the safety and trust in yourself to make active learning palatable. Then, it can take time to trust another person who tries to tell you something contrary to what you have already learned.

Think about this.

All your life you have learned the sky is blue. Right?

It's not.

I'm going to be quiet for a minute and let you think about that...

How did it feel to read "It's not" above? The truth, from an optical science point of view, is that the sky is every color except blue. For our everyday purposes, that is completely useless information—but it is still true. That feeling you had at reading it came from the redundant systems in your brain that are there to protect your learning and keep you efficient and safe. We will delve deeper into this as we progress, but we have to start there—understanding the power and trepidation involved in learning.

For our purposes here, it is sufficient to think in terms of safety and efficiency as main driving forces of our emotions and behavior. If we treat the brain as capable of more than this on its own, if we leave it in charge of our lives, we often run into trouble.

We are not our brains, though. Therefore, both those who provide and those who seek treatment benefit from a broader understanding of who we are as a whole. This understanding needs to prevail throughout the healing journey, and it starts with truly comprehending the process of therapy.

Sally Goes to the Doctor

Indulge me a moment here . . .

Imagine that Sally's knee, rather than her psyche, hurts. She tells her primary care physician about it and receives a referral to an orthopedic surgeon. Obediently, she schedules the appointment and shows up on time. After a lengthy wait in the lobby, she is called into the office, where she spends twenty minutes with this stranger. They do not ask about her homelife or spend much (if any) time at all learning about Sally as a person. The question, "How will this treatment affect your life?" is never asked. Instead, they probe for pertinent medical background, poke and prod her, and end the time with directions to return in a few weeks. Then, they will knock Sally out, cut her open, take things out of her, and replace them with a foreign body.

This, Sally will do (usually, without question).

Conversely, send Sally to the therapist with a heartache rather than a sore knee, and the story changes drastically. The therapist considerately and methodically spends weeks, or even months, trying to get to know and understand Sally and determine what effect treatment will have. Rather than being told what will happen, Sally is included in the formulation of the treatment at every point.

However, when the time comes to begin the emotional and psychological surgery, as it were, Sally resists the therapist's direction, vehemently at times.

What gives?

This is no slam on Sally at all. This is to be expected, as it is my belief Sally has a mental framework (or model) for what medical science will do with and for her, but not so with the process of therapy. This needs to change. Sally and those who seek help need to have a way to grasp what is happening in the recovery journey.

Therapeutic neuroscience can help.

What's the Catch?

As with anything, there are limitations to the ideas presented in this book. I will start with those.

Most of us are not neuroscientists. Even if we were, we would likely have specialized and not be versed in everything related to the science. We need to be aware of information deficits and honestly reply to concerns. Even so, we will not be able to answer all of our or others' questions.

This need not be problematic. As C. S. Lewis once said, "People ate their dinners and felt better long before the theory of vitamins was ever heard of . . ." (Lewis, 1952). People need not understand all the nooks and crannies to benefit from treatment. In fact, trying to understand too many details can derail progress. I have found it to be more valuable to understand analogies or "ways of thinking" than hard facts and data points. For everyday use, a practical direction rather than a true theoretical understanding is the key. This approach will satisfy most people.

You may occasionally encounter the person who will want more than you can give. In such cases, it may be beneficial to have a list of journal articles, prominent authors in the science, and books revealing more detail (such as those in the reference section of the appendix of this book).

In addition to the oversimplification issue, it is important to use and/or share only the information you have understood and thoroughly integrated yourself. Even as limited as our understanding is, those of you who grasp the gist of this book will likely know more on the topic than the majority of those with whom you interact. Overload will happen at times, so use wisdom in choosing what to convey. For those who teach, ask yourself, "What is the benefit of saying this?"

Finally, have you noticed how rapidly science and technology change? There are breakthroughs all the time. As soon as something is presented as a scientific fact, something else comes along to negate or expound on it in such a way as to change our basic understanding of it entirely. The breakneck speed of change can be maddening. This is why the use of concepts and analogies may be more beneficial than knowledge of pure scientific detail.

When all is said and done, the ability to separate brain and mind will be helpful to increase motivation and reduce shame for many people. Understanding this concept begins with developing a fuller picture of what it means to be a whole person.

Tips & Tricks (For the Journey of Recovery)

Media has much to say about neuroscience these days. Buzz-words abound! Take a minute to think about what you already know about the topic. Whether you are seeker or healer, this book may challenge you. Some information may contradict previous learning. It can be very helpful to approach new material as like a curious investigator rather than a deciding judge. When you find yourself reacting strongly to new information, consider doing one of the following:

- Write a pro and con list for adopting the new thought.
- Search for one other trusted source in support of the new thought.
- Ask yourself how life would be different if the thought was true.

Chapter Challenge Questions (Cortex Focus)

1. After reading this section, what do you feel is the most beneficial reason to incorporate neuroscience into daily therapeutic treatment and/or recovery practice?
2. What does "You are not your brain" mean to you? How would you know if you (or someone else) was acting *as*

if they were their brain? How would you explain this to someone else?

3. What do you think is meant by "whole person"?

4. What is one new thing you can do/think/teach/try with what you learned in this chapter?

Go Deeper (Somatic Focus)

1. **Journal Prompt (Choose one or both)**: When I cannot answer all the questions I am asked, I feel . . . When I learn something new in contradiction to what I have learned before, I . . .

2. **Mindfulness Activity**: Sit quietly in a place where you will not be disturbed. Take in two or three deep breaths at a slow pace. Mentally scan your body from head to toe. Using all your basic senses (sight, sound, taste, touch, and smell), notice the difference between your brain and the rest of your body. Do this a few minutes every day at least four times over the next week. Talk with someone or journal about what you discover.

CHAPTER TWO

Meet the Whole Person

One in Eighteen Billion

PRETEND YOU ARE standing in an empty room on the fifteenth floor of an office building in a very large, busy city. You peer out the window and see the masses moving about on the street below. Some mosey and some rush. They all come in different sizes, shapes, and colors. The perspectives and experiences of each vary enormously. Any ten of them are likely to have ten different views on the same topic. Think about this for a minute.

Now I have a question for you. Be honest with the answer. Have you ever been frustrated by another person?

If you are a human being, then of course you have!

Now for another question—why? What causes the frustration? Go ahead, put the book down and think about it. Be as honest as you can. No filtering. Do you find people stubborn? Slow or lazy? Unwilling to change? Do you feel unheard? Ineffective? Lost? Make a mental (or, better yet, written) list.

Consider your list. Were you able to find many valid and logical reasons to be disgruntled with other people at times?

Final question: What do you say to yourself about your frustration? Keep pondering. My guess is your answer will fit nicely into one of two categories—"others are the problem," or, "I am the problem."

Let's continue with the imagery above. As you stand watching out the window, you know there are over seven billion people on the planet right now. You ponder how many there have been and how many will be in the future. The total number, you realize, is prodigious—but to have something you can grasp, you settle on, say, eighteen billion.

Sit with that number for a minute. The average human lives around two and a half billion seconds. In other words, if you could say a person's name every second of your life, you would only be a tenth of the way done when you breathed your last.

Finally, consider this: In all of human history—past, present, and future, in all of those eighteen billion, there is . . .

One.

You.

Ever.

Let this thought sink in for a minute. Really. Stop reading and think about it.

Besides being breathtakingly beautiful, the uniqueness of each human being is astronomical.

"Hannah! Where are you going with all of this?" you ask.

Life and people are far more complex than we make them out to be in our everyday lives. That is where I'm going with all of this.

Return to the idea of being frustrated by others. Remember what I said at the start of this book, namely that the brain can be thought of as a binary, rule-based machine? This means we tend to be categorical (either you kept the rule or broke it; it's either this or that). If left in charge, the brain will provide drastically oversimplified analyses of most situations.

For example, all people are not idiots because they drive too fast, and "stupid" does not define you simply because you could not stop yourself from overindulging. We tend to mentally beat ourselves or others for not being good enough. In a world with this level of variation, what does "good enough" really mean anyway?

What if, instead of beating on ourselves (or others), we chose to celebrate the monumental number of times we actually get things right? Given what we are up against, we are crazy good at most of what we do. Seriously! Get yourself off the beat-myself-up road. When you find yourself hung up in such mental rhetoric, the brain is in the driver's seat, and you are too amazing to live in that manner.

I will say it again: You are more than your brain.

When you live otherwise, you become subject to making decisions on what I call "brain babble."

Brain Babble

Last year, I took a business trip to Lubbock, Texas. While driving there from Midland (no quick feat, mind you), I was caught in a heavy flash flood. It was terrifying. For a few rather tense moments, I thought I was a goner. Thankfully, a huge, white truck came along and led me out. After another hour or so on the road, I arrived on the outskirts of Lubbock near a university. One would think there would be ample provisions of food near a university, but could I locate any? Nope. (Sorry, Lubbockites.)

Finally, after still more driving, I found a catfish diner. I had never had catfish before. I bought a meal and eagerly took my fare back to the hotel so I could eat it and relax.

It tasted like mud.

Disappointed and tired, I heard my brain say, "Lubbock is awful!"

Now, wait just a minute. What?

I had spent all of one and a half hours in Lubbock out of my nearly fifty years of existence—how on earth could I have made such a sweeping determination so quickly?

Flash forward, and I am in Rochester, New York. It was dark, and the area where I parked was far from the hotel entrance. I was a bit nervous. As I walked, I passed a couple of bars and a restaurant with a flashing sign in the window with the word "catfish" on it. Upon seeing the sign, I heard my brain say, "Rochester is awful." (See? Not just Lubbock.)

Do you see the problem here?

Remember the brain's two primary goals? Yes! You got it: safety and efficiency. To achieve this, decisions must be made at a rapid pace. Therefore, the brain acts quite often as an anticipation engine. Associative and categorical by nature and necessity, the brain works mainly on triggers. It can be helpful to think of associations in the brain as consisting mostly of do and don't do, good and bad, safe and dangerous. In my case, feeling uncomfortable in my surroundings and the thought of unpalatable food categorized my entire experience into the "bad" category. Why? To keep me safe and to save time! Having those situations together created the thought, "Rochester is awful."

This is brain babble.

Let's take this further. What if I had taken those thoughts to be true? What if I was called on to return to Lubbock or Rochester? If I believed my brain babble, I might be unwilling to go and might miss out on a wonderful experience. The moral of the story? You can't believe everything your brain tells you.

If what we are learning from neuroscience is correct, then the workings of the mind and the brain are two separate things. The brain, then, is not the be-all, end-all it has been treated as in times past. Science says something more is at play.

This is curious. What do I mean?

What follows is this teacher's way of giving you an answer (with a little help from my friends—the authors listed in my references).

The Mind

According to the Merriam-Webster Dictionary, **psychology** is "the science of mind and behavior," yet the average mental–health care provider may not even know what the word "mind" truly means. They may, in fact, think mind and brain are synonymous and interchangeable. Most people walking down the street (and the media, and doctors, and the know-it-all guy next door) certainly speak as if this is the case.

In his work, Dr. Daniel Siegel substantiates this by reporting that throughout all his travels, and in quizzing nearly one hundred thousand psychiatrists and psychologists, he had not come across many (if any) who could even define the term "mind" (Siegel, 2010). What exactly is it, then? I think Siegel's definition is best:

> "The mind is an embodied and relational process that regulates the flow of energy and information" (Siegel, 2010).

This is abstract, to say the least. To understand this better, let's begin with the four-dimensional nature of the human.

The Four-Part Being

Consider the human to be a four-dimensional creature. Try not to be distracted by my word choice here. Speaking of all these aspects of a person as stemming from neuroscience is relatively novel. The language will stabilize as it is mulled and debated over time. I use the words I do simply to explain a concept.

To begin, consider the individual can be separated into three equally important parts: mind, body, and spirit. Then, the person themselves must be considered in relation to others—the social aspect. Hence, the four dimensions.

For our purposes, think of body, mind, and spirit as three elements of a system, analogous to an airplane. The plane itself is like the physical body, the pilot is the mind, and the character of the plane and its associated journey is the spirit. In this analogy, the brain is akin to the guidance system.

As with a plane, people cannot be thought of in isolation. We are all connected. Air traffic controllers are as important to the flight plan as the plane itself. We will only scratch the surface of this idea here, but I believe it is worth at least a surface discussion.

Consider the following three aspects of a person.

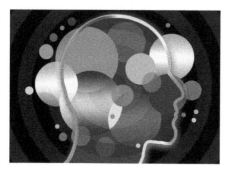

MIND. It can be useful to think of the mind as *that entity or process which uses* information from the brain, body, others/environment, and the big picture to create story and make decisions. This is analogous to the pilot using information from the engine, guidance system, air traffic controllers, and route to make decisions about how to interact with and/or drive the plane. In well-worn routes, autopilot can prevail. However, in new situations, in a storm, or if off course for some reason, the pilot must take charge and may even need to override the instruments. This analogy is limited but gives the idea.

BODY. It may seem odd to even define this term. Everyone knows what our body is—right? Sure—but it needs to be said simply and directly: The body is the physical [apparatus/vessel] that houses the blood, organs, and other structures that enable life-giving/life-continuing functions and allows us to interact with/sense our environments. The brain, then, is the organ within the skull that is linked to the rest of the body via the nervous system/spinal cord. It coordinates

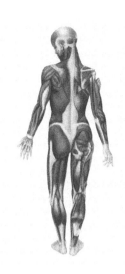

sensation, intellect, and nervous activity via trillions of neuron connections (more to come on this). The brain and body (guidance system and plane) are instruments with and within which the mind (pilot) and spirit (individual) create our unique journey and interact with and interpret the world around us.

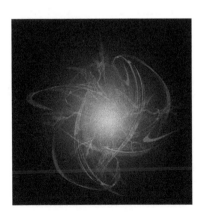

SPIRIT. This is a tricky one as there does not appear to be consensus as to the precise definition. Most definitions agree that the spirit is also "non-physical" and may include a person's nature, character, and/or "inner" or "true" self. As with the mind, the spirit is within us and between us, seeking to connect to something "greater than itself." Social connection and other spiritual practices (such as deep breathing, meditation, and prayer) are vital to health. These practices, if done mindfully, have been shown scientifically to positively affect the brain and are recognized as beneficial to both mind and body.

The concept of the separate nature of the mind and brain is abstract and complex. A helpful way to think of this may be to imagine the brain (guidance system) as a set of rules and algorithms whose job is to provide situational information. The mind (pilot) interprets this information and uses it to narrate life, make decisions, and adjust the system. The spirit, working in conjunction with the mind, draws from a myriad of factors, such as moral base, religious faith, character, social connection, life experience, and direction, to create the unique individual with their preferences and life goals.

Let's return to Dr. Siegel's definition of mind. It begins with the concept of the mind as embodied and relational. Recent advances in neuroscience (backed up by millennia of conventional wisdom) demonstrate that our minds extend outside of us to include others, so much so that our very brains and states of being can be altered by social experience. This refers to the fourth dimension of the person—their social connections—and it is a scientific notion! This has been addressed in depth in attachment theory, a model of psychological study and treatment that aims to improve connections between people. It has also been demonstrated scientifically with the identification of certain elements in our brains known as "mirror neurons."

Mirror neurons (which may reside in the inferior frontal cortex and superior parietal lobes of the brain) are a particular group of neurons that fire in response to what we see others do. (See the What Is Neuroplasticity section later in this book or the research study conducted by Giacomo Rizzolatti, MD, et al [1992], for more information on these types of neurons.) These neurons are what cause us to flinch when we see someone else fall.

Further, studies have shown that brains are changed, energized, and develop best in relation to others. Yes! Our brains need other brains to survive and thrive. This is stunning information. Connection is not simply something nice to have—it is an actual essential brain function.

This brings us to the second half of Siegel's definition: "to regulate the flow of information and energy." You wince when the other person falls; you do not then automatically fall down yourself. However, there may be occasions when your friend is hurting badly enough for you to feel as if the pain is your own. If your system is overwhelmed by others, then you need the mind to use what is received (or felt) to make changes in brain, behavior, and affect to manage the experience.

In the beginning, there is often no distinction between the brain and the mind. This is referred to as *cognitive fusion*. At this point, the guidance system is essentially stuck on autopilot. In this state of being, it will feel as if the plane and the pilot are one and the same. Autopilot serves an important purpose. It reduces fatigue and can be more accurate and speedier than the mind in certain instances. The pilot need not make any decisions or changes when all is running according to plan. However, when changes occur, there may be problems if the pilot is asleep.

The idea of brain being separate from mind is tough, I know. Chew on it for a while. More or less, happenings in the body, in the brain, and between people are not simple one- or two-step processes. They need to be coordinated and fit into a vastly intricate and multifarious picture. Before you run away screaming from the overload, check out the next section on the meaning of mental health.

What Is Mental Health?

If you have been totally wigged out by the utter complexity of the human system, never fear! Yes, we are all quite different, but we also have enough overlap to have guideposts to help us conceptualize the healing journey.

When walking the road of recovery, interpersonal neurobiology gives us two important mile markers of mental health: balance and integration.

Balance, for our purposes, can be thought of as a system whose components are in proper proportion such that the system is rendered stable. Balance does not mean all parts are equal. Think about work, for example. Few (if any) people need eight hours of work and eight hours of fun every day to have a fulfilling life.

I once knew a woman with a type-A personality who worked over one hundred hours a week in a high-stress job. However, she spent ninety minutes every week teaching small children to dance. The brief time she spent teaching balanced her entire system, and she felt strong and was able to consistently and happily perform at peak.

On the other hand, I have known those who worked only ten hours a week, but the work was so abhorrent to them they needed many, many more hours of play to feel balanced. In fact, there have been times when balance was unattainable because the work was too demeaning, strenuous, or boring.

The goal in recovery, then, is to figure out the combination of physical, emotional, mental, social, and spiritual acts needed to help a person remain steady and stable.

Integration, on the other hand, means all the balanced parts work well together. Perhaps Marty goes to therapy for a while and learns he has cognitive distortions. He learns to think healthier thoughts, but every time he speaks to someone about himself, he uses derogatory names and he avoids that which even hints at being outside his comfort zone. Can you see? Marty is not integrated.

Within the person themselves, it can be helpful to think in terms of components being aligned. We can see evidence of this alignment in what we think, say, and do. Concerning relationships, achieving interdependence is the goal. *Interdependence* is the highest level of maturity and is achieved when a person takes care of what they can on their own and knows when and how to ask for help with the rest. An adult relationship is not well integrated when there is over-dependence or an unhealthy level of independence. This book will not help you diagnose either of these states but hopefully will encourage you to be aware of their existence and meaning and to seek evaluation if needed.

There you have it. You are four-dimensional. Isn't that interesting? With the idea in mind of how this four-part system works together to create well-being, we can begin talk of the brain and body without confusing them with the system itself.

Tips & Tricks (For the Journey of Recovery)

When explaining the whole person to others, analogies (such as the airplane) are far more helpful than philosophical debates, overly scientific terminology, or other formal rhetoric. Have a discussion. Ask and answer questions. Admit when you do not know something. Do not presume anything. Stay open to different definitions. As long as the concept of a multifaceted person connected to other persons is conveyed, you're golden. When in doubt, return to the tips and tricks in chapter one.

Chapter Challenge Questions (Cortex Focus)

1. What does it mean to you to be "one in eighteen billion"? How does this change your view of yourself and/or others, if it does?
2. Explain the human being in your own terms.
3. How do you anticipate your clients (or others) will respond to this new information? What analogies will you use? What questions might they ask, and how will you respond?
4. What do you already know about the brain? Write down any words, phrases, or information you know.

Go Deeper (Somatic Focus)

1. **Expressive Arts**. Draw a picture of yourself in the world, yourself in your family, and/or just yourself. And/or write a song, poem, or story of the same. Set it aside. Come back in a few days and look at it. What do you notice?

2. **Mindfulness Activity**. Find a time and place where you can be uninterrupted. Then, find a picture of yourself when you were a different age, preferably a picture prompting pleasant feelings. Find a quiet place and set the picture in front of you. Using your imagination, remember the scene in vivid sensory detail. What did you notice through your skin, nose, ears, eyes, and taste? Remembering you are body, mind, spirit, and relationships, what would you like to say to the you in the picture? What do you think they would say in response? Have a conversation.

CHAPTER THREE

Therapeutic Neuroscience

THE TIME HAS finally come to learn about the brain and body itself. An exciting section for us science-y types. Without further delay, here we go!

Neuroplasticity—"It's All in Your Head"

Ever heard this saying? It is usually code for "Whatever is happening to you is made up," or worse, "You are crazy!" Pretty irritating phrase, isn't it? Take a look at this:

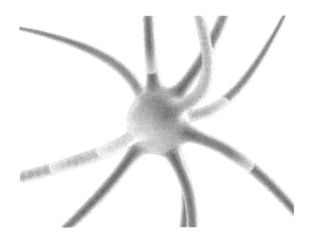

What is it? Is it a real thing? A neuron, you say?

Why yes, it is! And equally, it is a real thing. Someone may rightly say mental health disorders are "in your head" if they mean a chemical malfunction in the brain. However, it is incorrect to say mental illness is not real. Mental health issues are every bit as real as arthritis, diabetes, and cancer—and like them, are not character flaws.

While we are on the subject—what the heck is a neuron, and what does it do? The neuron is the basic building block of the mind-body-social communication system. The typical brain neuron has four main parts: dendrites, soma, axon, and synapse. The dendrites are the little tentacles attached to the cell body (soma). Neurons communicate via electricity and chemical messengers known as neurotransmitters. These chemicals pass through the dendrites, across the synaptic space, through the synapses, and then through the axon to the soma, where the process begins again as one neuron "talks" to another.

Neuronal firing in a healthy brain is not random but follows a certain pattern, depending on the specific communication. Lines of neuronal communication are known as neural pathways. When the same path of neurons fires repeatedly, this is known as the Hebbian principle, more commonly known from the statement "Neurons that fire together, wire together (Hebb, 1949)."

This is this basic process we now know makes it possible for both rigidity and flexibility in the brain—depending (at least in part) on whether the pilot (the mind) has any input or not. Left to its own devices, the brain will fire in comfortable, known patterns, as this is—you guessed it—efficient. However, there are times we need to alter the pattern to fit a change in the present moment. The fabulous news is that making these changes in neuron firing is possible and this change is known as *neuroplasticity*.

Brain Basics

To make sure we are all on the same page, here is some basic brain anatomy.

The human brain is made up of the brain stem, cerebellum, and four specialized regions called *lobes*. Each lobe has a right and left side separated by a membrane called the **corpus callosum**. Each portion of the brain consists of many smaller regions responsible for a multitude of specific tasks. However, for this discussion, only the primary functions for each major area will be presented.

Starting from the back and base of the skull, there is the brain stem and cerebellum.

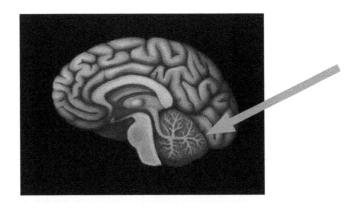

The **brain stem** is responsible for basic life functions, such as breathing, heart rate, and swallowing. Directly above the brain stem lies the **cerebellum**, which facilitates communication between the brain and the rest of the body. This part of the brain regulates movement in the body and processes input from our senses. Even lizards and hedgehogs have a brain stem and cerebellum.

Above the brain stem is the first major brain region, the *oc-*

cipital lobe. This area specializes in processing visual information. Moving from the lower back toward the front, the next set of lobes are the *temporal lobes*, which are positioned on both sides of the skull near each ear. These lobes process auditory information, organize the information with certain memory and time-related tags, and perform some language processing.

Next, at the top of the brain, are the *parietal lobes*. The motor cortex and major sensory processors of the brain are housed here. Finally, the forward-most region is known as the *frontal lobe*, which is the seat of awareness, executive functioning, judgment, and overall social behavior.

Region/Lobe of the Brain	Main Function
Brain Stem & Cerebellum	Basic Life Function & Communication between Brain & Body
Frontal Lobe	Cognitive Processing & Voluntary Movement
Occipital Lobe	Visual Processing
Parietal Lobe	Motor & Sensory Processing
Temporal Lobe	Language Processing & Certain Memory Processing

Thinking in terms of lobes can help us know which major function happens in which general region of the brain. However, there is another way to analyze brain structure. The brain can also be thought of as divided into three main parts, sometimes referred to as "the three brains" or "the triune brain." Unlike the lobes, which were described from the back forward, the three brains can be thought of as lower, central, and outer structures.

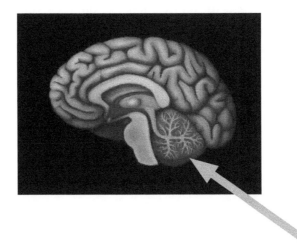

The first, or lower, brain consists of the brain stem and cerebellum. This region is referred to in many different ways, such as the **hindbrain** and the **reptilian** or **lizard brain.** This is due to its primary focus on baser life functions. Moving directly upward from there is the **central** or **mammalian brain.** This area is responsible for emotional and certain memory processing. The fight-or-flight response originates in this part of the brain.

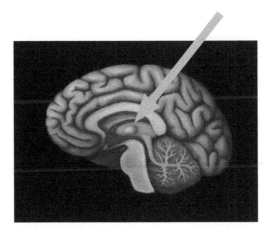

Finally, there is the entire outer section, the wrinkly part of the brain known as the *forebrain*, the **cortex**, or the **neocortex**. This is where thinking occurs.

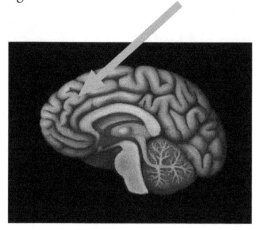

Within these regions are further areas of specialization particularly important in understanding the role of neuroscience in mental health practice. These are listed in the chart below with their associated primary functions.

Structure	Key Function
Amygdala	Warning System
Thalamus	Sensory & Motor Relay
Cortex	Thinking/Executive Function (in some areas)
Frontal Lobe	Executive Function & Social Rules
Hippocampus	Memory Storage

In the lower, central part of the brain is something known as the *amygdala*, often referred to as the "fire alarm" of the brain. Pay close attention to where it is: the lower, central part of the brain. Why is this important? Because the amygdala is not in the thinky part of the brain. Nope! By itself, the amygdala works only by association (or trigger), not by present moment detail. Can you already imagine how crucial this is?

Next, we have the *thalamus*. Notice where this is: the upper central part of the brain, close to the cortex but also not too far from the *limbic system*, the part of the brain responsible for fight or flight, as well as basic emotions and drives. You can think of the thalamus as Grand Central Station. This part of the brain controls motor relay. Everything comes into the thalamus first. The importance of this is monumental when it comes to anxiety—more on this concept later.

The *cortex* is the entire outer fold of the brain, from the frontal lobe all the way back to the occipital lobe. The cortex is where we think. Read that again. Do you see it? Yes! We think all over the higher regions of our brains! Not just in the conscious region. The frontal lobe houses all our social rules, and the area directly over the left eye (the dorsal-lateral prefrontal cortex) is the place of awareness and some higher executive functions. A lot of necessary work happens there, but thinking does occur in other places.

Finally, we have the *hippocampus*, one area of memory storage. Look at where this structure is in the brain—right next to our friend, the amygdala, which uses its proximity to tag memory with emotion.

What? Did I read you right?

Yes, you did! Memory can be tagged for retrieval by something other than words or even time! Remember the last time you ate something you did not like? What happened when you saw it again? You just knew you didn't like it, right? You may even have the emotion of repulsion come over you. When this occurs, it is a noticeable instance of the amygdala and hippocampus acting in cahoots. This will become very important for us later.

More on Neuroplasticity

Suppose you are in your car driving to work and you want a cup of coffee. After the conscious awareness (sometimes semiconscious) of wanting coffee occurs, it is unlikely you would ever consciously think, *Pull car over. Put on brake. Stop car. Put in park. Left arm, roll down window. Mouth, speak your order* . . . and so on. No. After the original decision to find coffee has been made, you somehow end up at the drive-through in front of your favorite java spot. Ever wonder how this happens?

Most likely, when you sought out and found coffee the first time, you had to be consciously aware of what you were doing. You had to decide on and find a place and maybe even think of how to make an order. Accomplishing the task required a particular set of neurons in your brain to fire. The next time you did the same task, found the same coffee in the same place, the identical set of neurons would have fired.

Usually, the first few times require some level of conscious input. However, over time, this same line of ignited neurons requires less and less conscious direction. Depending on the nature of what you are attempting to do, it can take some time to create a fixed firing pattern, but at some point, many of the repetitive actions in which we engage become completely nonconscious and unlikely to change without awareness and volition. This process—called *learning* or *habituation* (hmm, where have we seen that word before?)—is necessary, as it is the mechanism needed to create efficiency.

Neurons firing together in a line are called *neural pathways*. All the various structures and regions of the brain talk to each other via these pathways, which are made up of millions of *neural con-*

nections. In fact, a single neuron can have over ten thousand connections! Consider this next time you expect a change to happen quickly. Not only are we one in eighteen billion, but every thought or action could be one in trillions! Let yourself off the hook for expecting one-size-fits-all approaches to work!

Groups of neural pathways firing together frequently are referred to as **neural networks**. These networks can become hardwired. When this occurs, the resulting actions are usually nonconscious. This is where it can be a bit spooky sometimes. Imagine you are driving your normal route home. You are a bit perturbed because of something a coworker did. Mulling over it is taking all your concentration. The neural networks responsible for your ability to drive a car run automatically without your input. Suddenly, you arrive at your driveway, amazed you made it there so fast. Most likely, it took the same amount of time as usual, but because you were not paying attention, you did not notice.

I have a slightly off-topic question for you. Here goes: Have you ever said to yourself, "Why did I do that?" or "Why am I doing this?" What about, "Why am I doing this *again*?" These questions are indicative of times when you have noticed your brain mindlessly running the ship. Can you see the importance of engaging the mind? The hard fact is some neural pathways can be engaged and even solidified from the nonconscious area of our brains. Imagine the implications!

The significance of all this is that every thought we have and every action we take originates in the brain through neurons firing in increasingly predictable patterns.

Wait a minute . . . all this talk of neural pathways sounds like neuro-rigidity rather than neuroplasticity to me.

I hear you. Yes! Rigid responses are often the underlying issue when things go awry. This occurs most when we are cognitively fused and living on autopilot rather than engaging the mind.

Brain efficiency, then, can be both wonderfully helpful and, without mindfulness, frighteningly problematic. Just as breathing carries on without conscious thought but can be controlled if you choose, the same is true with some hardwired neural circuits. When working on routine tasks, the efficiency of an automatic system is desirable. However, when responding to variances in a rote manner rather than with flexibility, challenges arise. I'll say it again—the brain, albeit wondrous, can land a person in trouble when left to its own devices. Therefore, the mind is needed for momentary flexibility or to make neuroplastic adjustments in brain circuitry before returning to a habituated state.

Tips & Tricks (For the Journey of Recovery)

Attempting *cognitive defusion*, separating the brain and the mind, can be very difficult at first. You will initially need high levels of attention in the present moment to make changes. Eventually, your new skills and beliefs will integrate into the efficient system of the brain and become easier. In the beginning, however, it can be very helpful to:

1. **Choose one new skill or belief to focus on at a time**. Attempting to do too much at one time results in overload. Sometimes, less is more. This is one of those times.
2. **Allow yourself extra rest**. Staying at a heightened alert state taxes the awareness part of your brain. It is not unusual to feel more tired, restless, or even irritable when learning new skills. Allow yourself space to relax and take a few extra things off your plate if you can.
3. **Use your environment to prompt you**. It can reduce mental load to use something other than your brain to keep you on track. Develop a monitoring system to prompt you to use new behaviors, think new thoughts, and check in with yourself. For example, use sticky notes, pop-up notes on

your phone, or putting things in a particular place so you won't forget them.

Chapter Challenge Questions (Cortex Focus)

1. "There is freedom in knowing we humans are too astronomically complex for a one-size-fits-all approach." Do you agree with this statement? Is it a helpful thought? Why or why not?
2. What are the implications of neural pathways being created from the nonconscious regions in our brains?
3. What do you already know about structures and systems in the brain and body (such as the central nervous system)? Has what you know helped you in any way so far?

Go Deeper (Somatic Focus)

1. **SNAGing the brain**. Dr. Daniel Siegel has introduced the acronym SNAG as a way of increasing neuroplasticity (Siegel, 2010). SNAG stands for ***Stimulating Neuronal Activation and Growth***. Here are some ways to SNAG the brain:
   a. Aerobic exercise (twenty minutes should do it)
   b. Learning a new language
   c. Playing brain-based challenging games

CHAPTER FOUR

Pertinent Brain Structures, Processes & Functions

It's Easier to Balance Two

REMEMBER HOW BALANCE and integration are key markers of mental health? I think most people would agree balancing two is easier than three, four, or more. As further evidence of how wonderfully wired we are, a survey of the major systems we need to balance will show us each of them has precisely two parts.

The first set of two we will look at are the two sides (hemispheres) of the brain.

Right & Left Hemispheres: "Do You Have a Right Brain, Sir?"

For a few years, I ran an anxiety group in a partial-hospital program. Now and then, we would start the group out with a game wherein group members created a funny story by adding a silly sentence. Laughter temporarily cures anxiety and allows us a moment with a less tense body. However, one time, as the group played this game, we came to a particular group member who showed some resistance. They sat with their arms crossed and appeared to be holding their breath in a stature of defiance. Amused and a bit puzzled, I asked what the problem was.

"I have not worked so hard to come all this way to play games!" was their retort.

Understanding, I posed the question, "Do you have a right brain, my dear?"

You may have heard there is significance to the *hemispheres*. For years, I had them all mixed up. "The right brain, uh . . . umm . . . well, one of them is logic and one of them is art," is what I used to say when asked about them. Upon further study, I was appalled to realize no one had ever drilled deeper into this with me. This is not new news, folks! Someone should have told us! Thankfully, this information is finally reaching the people who need it. Better late than never, I suppose.

Anyhow, if you remember, the hemispheres are connected via a group of fibers known as the corpus callosum, which allow for communication between both sides. Brains can be (and often are) different, and we are oversimplifying—but for our purposes, this works. Concerning the hemispheres, there is significance to the functions of each one. Take a look.

LEFT BRAIN	RIGHT BRAIN
Analytical Thought	Intuitive Thought
Detail-oriented Perception	Holistic Perception
Ordered Sequencing	Random Sequencing
Rational Thought	Emotional Thought
Verbal Processing	Nonverbal Processing
Math	Writing & Expressive Arts
Logic	Imagination

Notice all the primary functions of the left side of the brain. Think of it as logical, linear, and linguistic. In other words, when you are speaking, doing math, and thinking about the order of events, neuronal networks are firing in the left side of the brain. The left brain is generally the source for worry (fear about the future) and rumination (constant repetition of negative thoughts in the brain).

We Westerners revere the left side of the brain. We want to measure and catalog everything to "prove" it. Knowledge, as it were, is king. If someone says, "I don't know," I imagine the next phrase will be—you guessed it!—"Google it!" We are meant to know all things at all times, and we are enamored by uber-left-brainedness.

Turn now to the functions of the right side of the brain, which is far more creative and flexible than the left. It is responsible for nonverbal communication, emotional processing, and holistic perception. When you exercise, use, or respond to nonverbal communication; imagine the big picture; or participate in expressive arts, the right side of the brain is engaged. The right side is the culprit when frightening mental images provoke panic.

As a general rule, we are not as amenable to the knowledge, or noetic function, of the more creative right side. *Noesis* (or *noetics*) is the Greek term for the deep knowing people have, without words or time attached. We do not know how we know some things; we just know we do. Have you ever met someone you know you know but cannot remember their name? Or have you ever entered a room and just felt off or really jazzed? How does this work? Another name for this is *intuition*, and it is absolutely a brain function and no less real than objectively measurable data. Both the left and right sides of the brain can learn something wrong, but our noetic understanding is right a lot (if not most) of the time!

Can you see the important distinction in the functions of the two hemispheres? Traditionally, modern psychotherapy makes use of only a portion of the left side of the brain. The problem, therefore, is that talking—especially abstractly—does not engage the whole brain. Let us explore both how to notice when there is left and right brain imbalance and how to manage it.

Hemispheres: Out of Balance?

At this point, I am wondering if you can already guess some signs a person is out of balance with respect to hemispheres. Most people have traits that indicate they favor a particular side. This, in and of itself, is not a problem. By saying "out of balance," I mean that the leanings cause noticeable difficulty in managing life, relationships, and/or work.

For example, you would expect a person who leaned more heavily to the left or the right to demonstrate certain perfectly acceptable traits. However, if the traits interfere with communication, cause anxiety or depression, or otherwise inhibit daily function, there is a problem.

Typical traits of those who are overly left-brained may include planning and scheduling rigidity, which is distressing to themselves, friends, or family; excessive analysis to the point of appearing unfeeling or unable to connect to others (always in their head); the inability to relate to the "irrationality" of emotions (finds them dumb); or difficulty picking up on subtle, nonverbal language (often calls themselves socially awkward). This is not an exhaustive list, but these are highly common. You can extrapolate from here.

The excessively-right-brained person may be someone who seems to have no sense of time. Though they often accomplish tasks they need to, they tend to put things off to the last minute. Over time, this may cause lingering stress and somatic symptoms. They tend to be artistic, creative, or kinesthetic and will prefer to perform these activities to the exclusion of more rigid work.

Both of these presentations have strong positive qualities as well. Left-brained leaners tend to be efficient and logical, and they enjoy solving problems. They are excellent planners and are not rattled easily if they can see a clear solution. Those who favor the right brain are emotionally open and sensitive (if allowed to be themselves), creative, innovative, and out-of-the-box thinkers.

Remember, the goal is balance, which does not mean equal in amount. As mentioned, a leaning one way or the other is perfectly healthy. Even so, many of the left-brain-dominant people who come to treatment for anxiety disorders are described by their friends (and even themselves, at times) as too detached. Those who are right-brain-dominant are told they are too impulsive.

When dealing with a person who leans heavily into their right brain, cognitive behavioral therapy is the approach of choice, as skills for structuring thinking and measuring experience can be helpful. As an entire section is dedicated to CBT later, the focus here will be addressing those who lean too far into left-brain function. It is important to get them out of their heads and into their body, emotions, and environment. To that end, somatic-emotive (or body-and-emotion-based) treatment strategies are helpful. Thankfully, these have begun to proliferate as the science has continued to confirm the importance of addressing these hidden-in-plain-sight aspects of ourselves. These techniques are designed to pull the over-thinker out of their head and back in touch with their body and surroundings. Here are a couple to consider:[1]

Art Therapy

Art therapy is a robust, therapeutically relevant treatment, as it taps into our struggles with semantic expression. Art therapy may include drawing, coloring, working with clay, creating collages, and using shape, color, and perspective to describe feelings, thoughts, memories, experiences, and actions. Some counselors specialize in this type of treatment. For those of us who wish to

---

[1] Please do not try any of the techniques in this book without a firm understanding. These examples are simply for illustrative purposes.

utilize some basic concepts, there are many art therapy books filled with basic exercises. One example is *250 Brief, Creative & Practical Art Therapy Techniques: A Guide for Clinicians and Clients*, by Susan I. Buchalter.

Body Scan

Some people might act surprised if you remind them of the body dangling off that head of theirs! Some people are simply not connected well to themselves. A body scan allows a person to consciously, and mindfully (over time), attend to their bodies. The end goal is relaxation, but this rarely happens in the beginning. In fact, anxiety can worsen at first. If we have been stuck inside our heads, we can be oblivious to what is happening in the body. After all, if it is moving and breathing, it is fine, right?

Nope.

A body scan begins by having the person relax, center their breathing, and then, guided by the therapist, attend to each major area of their body. Memories are stored in the body and can be revealed by a body scan. Therefore, I suggest if you have never done a body scan before with a particular client, you always start with the feet. Start with the feet because feet are grounded, and feet are not commonly abused. It gives the client at least a few minutes of relative calm experience, as a body scan can be unpleasant in places at first.

It can be helpful to use an outline of a human figure to capture information during body scans.[2] If you notice a twitch or grimace or even an uptick in breathing or shaking or bouncing a leg, place a check mark in the area of the body in which it occurs. After the scan is done, you can check back to see if there is any pain, discomfort, or fearful memories associated with a particular part of the body.

When you begin using this tool, start with a general body scan,

---

[2] For more examples and related worksheets, see https://bit.ly/3cutW0W.

scripts for which can be easily found with an online search. Over time you can be creative. One instance of this for me is something I call a Gratitude Scan (see the link to worksheets). Gratitude can be a difficult topic for some people. Many who struggle with depression have been shamed with statements such as "You have so much; you should just be thankful." In other words, "Why are you sad? You have so many things."

Can you see the problem with this line of thinking?

As you will clearly understand by the end of this section (if you don't already), in times of trouble, the brain is deficit oriented. Remember: safety and efficiency. As a general rule, we do not need to be on the lookout for happiness and joy in the same way we do for trouble and sorrow. Therefore, gratitude brings our assets to the awareness of the brain. The Gratitude Scan may help those who struggle with overall positivity or body-image issues to realize their assets as well as deficits, which can increase hope.

In case you would like to keep learning about other somatic-emotive techniques, they include group therapy, guided imagery, narrative therapy, psychodrama, yoga, meditation and mindfulness, play therapy, equine therapy, emotion-focused and emotional-freedom techniques, and the use of Polyvagal and attachment theory. I encourage you to build your repertoire of skills or to connect with other providers who practice any of these so you may make referrals. There is no shame in sharing!

Regulatory Systems: Two Sides of the Same Coin

In keeping with the theme of balance, just as there were two sides to the brain, there are also two major regulatory systems. These two systems are divisions of the autonomic nervous system (ANS), which means they are largely (but thankfully, not entirely) outside of our conscious control. They are the *sympathetic* and *parasympathetic systems*. You may have heard of these. Do you know what they do? If not, you are not alone. Most of us learned about these in college, but with no practical application, the information faded away.

The sympathetic system is responsible for the activation and acceleration of body systems—in other words, fight or flight. The parasympathetic system inhibits and slows down bodily functions, also referred to as "rest and digest." If a person leans too much into the sympathetic system, they are **up-regulated** and need to calm themselves to find balance. Too much activation of the parasympathetic system results in **down-regulation**, which requires behavioral activation to find equilibrium.

Take a minute, if you can right now, and find your pulse. Once you do, take some slow, deep breaths.

What do you notice?

When you breathe in, your heart rate often increases. When you breathe out, it decreases. In other words, if you are breathing in and out at a regular, calm, and normal pace, then your regulation systems are likely balanced. Breathing in activates just enough fight-or-flight to get us going, while breathing out calms us enough to not take off like a rocket at every moment. It's like magic! The body knows what it needs! Amazing, isn't it?

A question though. How do anxious people breathe? Right. Shallow, fast, and/or they may even hold their breath. Likewise, how do depressed folks breathe? Sigh . . . very, v e r y slowly. Think about this. By looking at the physical body, you can think of anxiety and depression as two sides to the same coin! Anxiety results in an up-regulation, and depression throws people into down-regulation.

For more insight, look at the following chart.

Sympathetic ("Fight or Flight")	Parasympathetic ("Rest & Digest")
✓ Excites ✓ Prompts increased output of energy ✓ Up Regulation: Dominant for terror, rage, excitement, elation ✓ Focus: Needs OUTSIDE the body	✓ Inhibits ✓ Prompts functions of growth and restoration ✓ Down Regulation: Dominant for shame, disgust, hopelessness, despair, detachment ✓ Focus: Needs INSIDE the body

The sympathetic nervous system, when activated, fills us with energy to keep us active and safe. The initiation of the more intense fight-or-flight response is uber fast and, therefore, essentially automatic. We do not ask for it, and it happens without our conscious will or permission.

This level of efficiency is necessary and helpful in moments when we are faced with life-threatening situations. However, when erroneously charged or put in overdrive, our brain filters become dominant for terror, rage, excitement, or elation. Take all of this in . . . our *brains* are dominant for this—not our *characters*. Character certainly has a place in our behaviors, but it is more the reaction to and not the source of the problem.

The hope is we notice an uptick in sympathetic activation at lower states—in anger, anxiety, surprise, and arousal. However, in times of more intense stress, you are not flawed, broken, or otherwise defective if you resort to these more forceful states of being. The goal would be not to reach these levels of stimulation, but if it happens without mindful awareness, then all people will likely end up in one of these emotional states.

When up-regulated, the brain is focused outward on the dangers in our environment. This is why it is crucial for those around an overly activated person to remain calm and reflect safety. Attempting to argue with someone who is up-regulated will only result in perpetuating irrationalities. The person may say and do things they would not normally say or do at other times. Here is an example:

> Joey had had enough. Despite being one of the most productive people on his team, he never felt appreciated, and others often guilted him into doing their work. Today had been the worst to date. Already at his limit, there was still the rough commute home. At least at home he could relax and let go for a few hours. Or so he thought.
>
> When Joey arrived home, his wife was sitting in the living room waiting for him. He had promised he would pay a particular bill, and he had forgotten. Her confrontation was too much. He was not in the mood. He asked to discuss it later, but she was unrelenting. Just wanting to be left alone to process, and knowing her tenuous relationship with her domineering mother, Joey shouted, "You're just like your mother! You push and you push, and you never let go!"
>
> Shocked and upset by his use of this pain point against her, Joey's wife stopped talking, went to the bedroom, slammed the door, and began to cry. Now there was an entirely new problem brewing. Joey did not mean what he said. He had never seen any similarity between his wife and her mother. He wondered why he had said it. Would she ever believe he did not mean it?

As you can see, this is an example of an up-regulated person, nonconsciously focused on the dangers of the environment, tagging a generally safe person as the enemy. In so doing, he pulled out the big guns and went for sore spots in her heart—not because he meant what he said, but simply because a part of him knew it would make her go away and leave him alone.

Remember, social rules are stored in both conscious and non-conscious areas of the brain. Our powerful forebrains, in wanting to help us, may actually cause us problems when outdated, junk, or corrupted files are pulled out for defense. If we can separate our characters from our biology and recognize when others are tiptoe-ing into irrational territory, we may save a lot of pain and misunderstanding.

What about the parasympathetic system? This is the part of the ANS responsible for relaxation and calm. As you can see from the chart, this system inhibits us and provides for restoration and growth. Many of us know highly anxious people who report an inability to relax. This is problematic and results in chronic up-regulation.

However, some people are too often or too intensely down-regulated. The lower-level activation of this system, sadness, is a healthy emotion necessary for a full life. Have you seen the Pixar movie *Inside Out*? It is a wonderful and remarkably accurate description of how emotions develop and work. Sadness, one of the characters, keeps falling in a puddle of her own tears and says, "Crying helps me slow down and obsess over the weight of life's problems." Her statement is brilliant!

Oh, if we could only fully grasp this concept! Sadness *does not* have to lead to excessive down-regulation. If we can allow ourselves to notice, feel, and grieve our losses, and if we can admit we need to feel purposeful and connected to life and others, then our griefs may heal and there may be less clinical depression. You might wonder why the brain would try to point out all the negative? It is not to make us own these things as if they were our just deserts—it is an attempt to force us to stop and address the causal issues.

When our losses and unfulfillment are not dealt with over time, we may end up with brains dominant for shame, disgust, hope-lessness, despair, and detachment. Prolonged down-regulation can result in clinical depression. Again, this begins as a function of our brains, *not our personalities*. In down-regulation, the motivational and reward centers of the brain are impaired. This causes a person to focus excessively on the needs of their own body, leaving them with little-to-no sense of connection, purpose, or joy. This contrib-utes to the "poor me" mentality many depressed people share. It makes sense though. I don't know about you, but I would be (and certainly was) pretty pitiful when feeling disconnected from life and depressed.

When looking at the system as a whole, whereas the sympa-thetic system is activated without our input, the magic of the para-sympathetic system is our ability to intentionally use it to reduce over-activation. Imagine walking your dog. Your neighbor calls to you from their house, and as you turn to greet them, you acciden-tally let go of the leash. Off Fee-Fee goes at a pretty good clip. Not wanting to lose your best friend, you take off after her. You run at (your) top speed for two solid minutes. Once you catch up to the little bugger, you find yourself breathing so hard you have spots before your eyes.

At times of stress, such as chasing Fee-Fee, if you use the para-sympathetic system and work to slow and deepen your breathing, you will find you are likely able to rebalance your system on your own. This takes practice, but thankfully, the same method can work for anxiety attacks and panic.

This is an overview of the state of imbalance in these systems. Next, let's look at some specific examples of how to restore stability.

Regulation Systems: Out of Balance?

Understanding these regulatory systems is of great benefit in mental health treatment. All aspects of our beings—mind, body, spirit, and social—play a role in mental illness. It is not only physical. In other words, simply breathing regularly will not cure anxiety or depression. However, starting with the physical may provide a safer inroad into treatment. People do not feel as much shame when they realize their reactions have a biological rather than personal origin.

As symptoms go, anxiety and mania involve up-regulation, and depression and lack of motivation indicate down-regulation. The question, then, is what do you do in either case?

Let'sstartfirstwiththatpersonwhotalksnon-stopnoteventakingabreaththeywanttotell youtheirwholelifestoryandyoucanbarelykeepup.

Whew! What?

You know—people with pressured speech who talk nonstop. Try as you might, you cannot get a word in edgewise. How do you usually feel in the presence of such agitation? If you are like most people, you feel a bit wound up too. You can thank the mirror neurons for this ability. You can also credit them for proving that we are, indeed, connected, social creatures.

Activating the parasympathetic system can be helpful here. If a person in therapy is talking with pressured speech, one useful technique is to get their attention and stop them. Have them join you in a deep breath and explain to them that their system may be out of balance. Then ask them, while speaking, to tap each finger on their hand with their thumb and allow only one word per tap to slow the pace down.

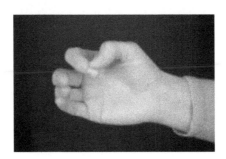

Have them continue this as long as necessary to reduce activation. If they go back to pressured speech, you can model the hand movements without interrupting them. You can do this throughout the session to keep returning them to a lower level of activation.

If they cannot use their hands in this manner, or if you are working in a group, you might try using a metronome instead. You can buy a physical one or find an app for them online. Use wisdom. This method works best at the onset of symptoms and may not be as effective if the person is in full mania or panic or has some fear related to the exercise.

Another way to adjust a hyped-up regulatory system is deep, controlled breathing. Most therapists have heard of, and may even teach, one method of this called diaphragmatic breathing. **Diaphragmatic breathing** is a specialized way to slow breathing. Another name for this is belly breathing. However, those who have a history of rapid or shallow breathing or those who tend to hold their breath may experience dizziness, nausea, or even fainting (syncope) when introduced to this type of breathing. To fully learn the mechanics of proper breathing, consider referring to a yoga instructor. Yoga is an evidence-based practice that engages all four dimensions of a person, calming mind and body and encouraging spiritual and social connections.

When working with a down-regulated system, a focus on engaging the sympathetic system via "behavioral activation" may be fruitful. Most clinicians use this method regularly. However, the problem is many have not known the biological reason behind it. Therefore, it can be packaged in such a way as to feel demeaning to the depressed person. I can remember, for example, having therapists who told me I needed to get out and exercise and interact with others more. I distinctly remember thinking they were telling me, "Get off your backside, you lazy bum!" I do not think I am the only one who ever thought this after such a directive.

The good news is, research has shown that only twenty minutes of aerobic exercise is enough to decrease amygdala activation (Johnsgard, 2004). For some people, this decrease can last for two days! While the goal is twenty minutes of heart-pumping movement, it is not the first step. The way I typically approach a depressed client is to teach them about these two biological systems and to let them know theirs is out of balance. To reignite it, I tell them to "make friends with movement." I do not say exercise. This is a scary and sometimes shaming word.

The benefit of working with the body first, besides decreasing shame, is in capitalizing on the quick changes that occur in the person's body. Reducing adrenaline and cortisol or increasing your heart rate will naturally result in a relatively rapid feel-better state. Not only will this improve their outlook, but it could have the extra added benefit of making a therapist look like a pretty smart cookie (if not an outright miracle worker).

Once people have noticed the benefits of movement, graduate them to higher and higher intensities. Go out for a walk or encourage them to start a mild yoga routine. Yoga is one of those activities with the ability to properly engage both regulatory systems while also incorporating breathing and movement. For anxious people, it can provide a calming release. For those with depression, it can be a gentle way to up the ante in an exercise routine.

Risks & Limitations.

All techniques are limited by scope and particular area of practice. Be mindful of your and the client's skill level before attempting a technique. Make sure you fully understand the mechanism of how it works and ensure they recognize the symptoms a given technique addresses. Finally, make sure anyone you work with is cleared medically, if applicable.

Processing Systems: Take It from the Top . . . or Bottom?

Two sides of the brain, two regulatory systems, and now—two mental processing systems!

As we live our lives, our brains take in stimulation from our surroundings and from within our bodies and process it into usable bits of information. Brain processing is not localized to only within our skulls. It involves a stimulus, emotions, body responses, cognition, and social and environmental cuing. These processing systems are referred to as top-down and bottom-up processing.

Top-down processing (or front-to-back/frontal-to-occipital-lobe processing) occurs as stimulation in the environment passes first through the frontal lobe (where rules and previous learning are activated). In other words, we apply thinking and already learned "rules" to what we perceive. By using information and understanding we already have, we make sense of or add meaning to what we see and experience. See the following example of top-down processing.

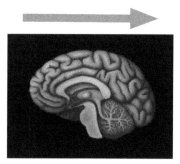

Wehn unisg a top-dwnn psrocses, you wlil be albe to urndstnad wrods taht are a ttoal mses, but hvae the smae nmrber of lteters and the frist and lsat letetr in the porepr pclae.

With something like this, you already know all the words, the syntax, and at least some of the context cues. Therefore, the perception of the words is made understandable by language rules you've already learned. As opposed to being able to understand, say:

Fgodaok, hgoy nem tduod ellvonasi ezt!

. . . which is the same idea as above but using Hungarian instead of English. Unless you speak Hungarian, you likely could not read the sentence. Therefore, *cognition drives perception*, and we experience what we expect to experience. In colloquial terms, we have bias or preconceived notions.

Suppose Margaret grew up in a house full of psychologists. After a breakup in high school, she saw a counselor for a while, and it really helped. If she saw a counselor later in life, she would likely walk in the door expecting success and would probably experience it.

Then there's Jim. He grew up in a critical family where he was teased for showing any emotion at all. No one ever offered support, and he was taught he needed to "man up." Jim's girlfriend notices he is often angry and may be depressed. She urges him to see a counselor. Jim's friend Edgar went to a counselor and did not improve. Jim has seen many derogatory television shows and read many negative media reports about counseling. He has been left with the belief there is not much use in trying it. Jim will likely resist going, and if he does go (to get the girlfriend off his back), he will probably go through the motions and stop after a while. Essentially, he will not expect to receive help from the process, and therefore, he won't.

There are many dynamics at play here. Jim has many rules in his brain. If violated, the result will be feelings of anxiety and guilt. As you can well imagine, most people will do anything to avoid these emotions. There is a lot stacked against him. His own family-of-origin experience taught him expressing emotion is wrong—

rule number one. Counseling is all about expressing emotion. Doing so will feel improper to Jim.

Jim has also never seen anyone close to him have success with counseling. Rule number two is, "Counseling does not work because it has not worked for my friends." This may even yield another rule: "It is not a good idea to find success with something my friends could not do." Rules such as these add brain filters or cause us to justify not practicing skills, and a whole host of other defensive actions.

People like Jim can overcome a negative bias. Maybe a new friend has a resounding success in counseling. Perhaps they try self-help books to open their mind to new possibilities. A faith experience can help. Or they might find a counselor who knows how to slip past a bias by listening carefully to their thoughts about counseling and pointing out how they work differently.

Alternatively, managing input in a more back-to-front/occipital-to-frontal-lobe manner is known as ***bottom-up processing***. This is a more holistic form of processing wherein the brain takes in stimulation from the environment first in the sensory part of the brain. As with the right brain, bottom-up is the type of processing most active in intuition and/or "gut feeling." Understanding this concept is a bit more difficult, as it is not possible to replicate a sense of something on a two-dimensional page. Bottom-up processing, over time, results in sensation driving cognition. Here is an example to make this idea clearer.

> Shelly was uncomfortable. She could not say why. She just did not feel right. It was the first day of class, and it was only ten minutes in when she had a powerful urge to run out of the room. Thankful she had found a seat in the back, she gathered all her belongings and left quickly and inconspicuously.
>
> Once home, Shelly called her friend Lyla and told her about the incident. "I'm not ever going back there!

Something is wrong!" she said with full conviction. Lyla asked many questions to try to determine what the problem was, but Shelly had no answer. This struck Lyla as odd, and she encouraged Shelly to return to see if anything changed. She even offered to come with her. Shelly resisted, believing something bad would happen if she returned.

This would be an example of when a bottom-up process *creates a cognition or drives a decision-making process.* As emotions are often strong and meant to push us in particular directions, it can be very difficult to change the mind of a person with a strong feeling about something. Taking small steps toward the feared or uncomfortable task or situation, tying the experience to another time when there was a success, or exposure therapy may be beneficial in moving a person through an uncomfortable feeling.

Processing Systems: Out of Balance?

What are signals that a person may have an imbalance in top-down processing? Look for people who know everything already, are cognitively biased and not easily talked out of their erroneous thoughts, and who struggle to dig into their intuition. For them, somatic/emotive techniques that help them connect internally may be of benefit. It is also very important to build rapport and truly listen to even highly irrational content, as it gives insight into possible origins.

Cognitive Behavioral Therapy (CBT) techniques and mindfulness, which may be defined as *nonjudgmental* awareness in the present moment with all senses, may be helpful techniques for those who are overly sensitive feelers. Take the person who has had some physical illness in the past who "just knows" they will be sick again. Living life in the current moment, as opposed to the feared future, is often safer for these people.

Remember our stuffy group memeber from the beginning of the chapter? Thankfully, they eventually learned to loosen up and play. In fact, by the end of his few weeks in the hospital, they had a renewed spring in their step, and had even reconnected with estranged family members! The moral of the story for this chapter is balance. Learn to find ways to notice when you or those with whom you work are out of balance. Our systems have the awesome ability to take care of us when allowed or taught to do so. Capitalize on this, and like the stuffy-turned-happy man, you may find the method you need to start someone on the road to healing.

Tips & Tricks (For the Journey of Recovery)

Balance is important in all areas of life for all people. Not everyone finds balance in the same way. On a macro level, your interactions with others (relationships and work, for example) need to be in balance. Within you, on a micro level, your body and brain also require equilibrium. Have a plan of action to cover all important areas of your life: mind, body, spirit, and social life. Consider writing a plan and hanging it somewhere you can see it often. Add a friend's phone number or the name of someone you admire for those moments when you want to talk yourself through steps you need for balance.

Chapter Challenge Questions (Cortex Focus)

1. What is it like for you to know that not all thinking happens in the conscious part of the brain?
2. What kind of healing work have you done that does not involve simply talking? (Examples: art or play therapy, group therapy, body scans . . . what else?)
3. How did you feel about these experiential modalities before reading this chapter? Did anything change? If so, what, how, and why do you think?
4. In down-regulation, the brain highlights shame, disgust,

hopelessness, despair, and detachment. If the point of this is to encourage us to notice these conditions and address them, can you think of one example of each and how you would tackle it?

Go Deeper (Somatic Focus)

1. Mindfulness Activity.
   a. **Left/Right Brain Balance**: Try a body scan of your choice.
   b. **Sympathetic/Parasympathetic Balance:** Find a place where you will not be interrupted. Sit in a comfortable position. Perform deep, diaphragmatic breathing for at least five to ten minutes. Focus your mind on your breathing. Use all your senses. Consider playing some calming music, lighting a rejuvenating scent in the room, or perhaps having a few sips of herbal tea before you start. Sit on a soft cushion and/or wear soft and comfortable clothing, and either close your eyes and create images in your mind or have something beautiful to look at throughout the meditation.
   c. **Top-Down/Bottom-Up Balance:** Focused meditation can access both cognitive and somatic functions. In meditation, the left brain has words on which to focus and the right brain notices breathing, beauty, gratitude, or other somatic-based concepts. Try a "Lovingkindness" meditation (see https://ggia.berkeley.edu/practice/loving_kindness_meditation for an example).

CHAPTER FIVE

Do You Remember?

A H MEMORY . . . THE malefactor in a great deal of mental health issues. The full treatment of memory is way beyond the scope of this book, but I want to highlight a few interesting points.

What *Do* You Remember?

Memory can be thought of as the encoding and storage of internal and external stimuli and experience. What does it mean to encode? This is what we do to "tag" a memory with a retrieval system. It is context-driven. For example, most people would say the word "please" is a nice word. We teach the little kiddies to say it, after all. However, I lived many years in India, and in the region in which I lived, "please" among friends is considered rude! Yes. Really.

For my friends in India, "please" and "thank you" were thought to create distance between people. A saying I often heard was, "Please and thank you are for the queen and the boss!" Many times, I was reprimanded for using these words. It was baffling at first. Being reprimanded (gently, albeit) for using words I had been taught were polite my whole life was jarring.

Back to our point: if I encoded a request, it would go something like, "Priti, could you please hand me that file?" To which Priti would respond, "Stop that! We're friends!" Likewise, when Priti encoded a request, it went something like, "Give me that file," to which I often recoiled, feeling bossed or scolded. For the first several months, I felt as if people around me were rude and brash.

However, over time, I realized dropping the formalities, for them, brought me closer. It was a compliment. Once I mindfully reminded myself enough times, it became comfortable, and I even felt odd when someone said please. You can imagine how I was when I came back to the US!

Everyone's encoding system has slight-to-great variations, depending on the commonalities of context and culture. Twins growing up in the same family will encode things differently. Understanding this, it is important to realize it is not our job as counselors and caregivers to download our encoding system into anyone else. As so eloquently stated in the famous book *7 Habits of Highly Effective People*, Stephen Covey says, "First understand, then seek to be understood" (Covey, 1994).

True or False?

Memory, then, is about taking in information about our experiences, but encoding and other factors can complicate matters. Sadly, we spend a lot of our time mining memory in ineffectual ways. To understand this, let's play a game. See if you can pass the following memory quiz:

Statement	True or False
We are always conscious of our memories	
We accurately remember our experiences	
Memory is like a puzzle—it comes in pieces	
Memories come to us in an orderly fashion	
The memory of past events can affect future function	
Memories are primarily located in one area of the brain	
Memories are only constructed by external factors	
Memories can be changed and refiled	

How do you think you did? Let's take these one at a time.

We are always conscious of our memories. *False*

Much of our memory has to do with how we do routine things, such as walk or talk, so there is no particular semantic or emotional tag for these. This type of memory has not been tagged for easy or conscious retrieval. Therefore, we are not aware of all memory. Think, for example, of the time you asked your fidgety client what was upsetting them, and they said they did not know. In such a case, their body knew, but their conscious mind did not.

We accurately remember our experiences. *False*

What did you do for your last birthday? What about Christmas? Try to remember. What details come to mind? If your friend asks you, you may remember cake and presents. If your coworker asks, you may remember you took the day off or had to work. Depending on the context in which something is recalled, the memory can change. In addition, our likes, dislikes, perceptions, and preferences can influence memory. If your favorite color is red, then you may remember a red boat on the fun trip you took last summer, only to be surprised to find a picture of a yellow boat.

Memories are like puzzles—they come in pieces. *True*

Return to the remembrance of your last birthday or Christmas. As you think about it, as you delve deeper into the memory, incorporating sensory information, you remember more and more. This is because memory is tagged and stored differently in various parts of the brain. Some memories are tagged with language-based recall mechanisms (semantics), and others are sensory or emotion-based. This is why a trauma survivor may remember a clock hanging on the wall but not the assailant's face at first. Sensory-based, emotional memory may be stronger in some senses than word-based (see explicit versus implicit memory below for more).

Memory comes to us in an orderly fashion. *False*

Memory retrieval changes depending on several factors, such as context, state of mind, and who is asking. As mentioned above, if your mother asks you how your birthday was, a whole slew of memories comes to mind without any conscious input. If, however, your boss asks you how your birthday was, a whole set of different memories will come all on their own. This often has to do with the way social or procedural rules dictate how our brains function. Interesting, isn't it?

The memory of past events can affect future function. *True*

Memory is tagged and stored the way it is to make our ability to forecast and react appropriately to the myriad of experiences we face every day safe and efficient. Think about it. It is important to know this is not always a logical process when the amygdala is involved. Imagine a child petting a dog. Their mom comes and smacks them on the head, scolding, "You should have been in an hour ago!" From then on, the child could be afraid of dogs. Not because the dog hurt them, but because playing with the dog was associated with the slap. After the incident, when the child wanders in the neighborhood, they may stay away from the dog's house without even being aware of their actions.

Memories are primarily located in one area of the brain. *False*

Memories can be stored and tagged in various areas of the brain. I will say more about this in a minute, but the location and tagging system matter. Memories stored in the left part of the cortex, for instance, may have time tags, while those memories tagged with emotion in the hippocampus may not. Can you imagine the implications of this?

Memories are only constructed by external factors. *False*

Another important consideration—memory can be constructed by our internal states. This is why two people doing the same activity could remember it differently. You and your best friend could go to a party with twenty-three other people. Twenty-one of them could talk to both of you. However, if the one person you most wanted to talk to didn't approach you, your brain could say to yourself at the end of the night, "No one talked to me at the party." This could become your memory. Imagine what your friend might say to this!

Memories can be changed and refiled. *True*

Hallelujah! This is often the task of healing.

What do I mean?

Have you ever had an experience of something unpleasant, say arriving late to someone's house because the person driving you was going way too slow? As you approach your house and contemplate the ride home, you may feel unhappy. Imagine as you enter the house you find out you were delayed on purpose because it was a surprise party for you. The moment you realize the reason for the delay, the memory of your ride home becomes more pleasant and positive.

The experience of a memory can change once seen from a different perspective. Of course, this process can be corrupted if someone attempts to replace a healthy memory with an unhealthy one. However, if you are on the road to recovery with a well-trained guide, the likelihood of false or erroneous memory creation is low. Their goal will be to use this key to help in your recovery.

Memory in the Mind versus the Brain

You have seen that memory may not be all you thought it was. We remember things, surely—but not always accurately, consciously, or in an orderly fashion. What, then, is the purpose of memory? Here is where one must separate the brain and the mind.

In the brain, memory is for safety and efficiency, which means memory is for *the future*. Most of your brain can be thought of as an anticipation or solution engine. What this means is your brain spends a great deal of time attempting to analyze your internal and external worlds to anticipate and prepare for what comes next. The more the brain and body can do on autopilot, the less fuel and energy used and the more likely the resources needed to watch out for problems will be there.

Think of the mind as the nostalgic part. The mind is the storyteller. It weaves bits and pieces together into a coherent whole. When under extreme stress, the brain's resources are narrowed to focus on whatever will keep the person alive. In those harrowing moments during an assault, something seemingly irrational could actually provide a focal point for concentration, thereby keeping us disconnected from harm and alive. It can take time for the neurochemicals elicited in such a situation to abate. Over time, the mind will retrieve and weave together a more coherent story.

Meeting the Inner Child

You now know you can retrieve, modify, and refile memories. It is not an easy process, and it involves reaching into the implicit storage systems, recovering fearful memories, and using explicit systems to add context, semantic understanding, and time tags. Think of the implications this process has on relationship issues and trauma. The truth for most of us is, without mindful awareness, we walk around in grown-up bodies with inner children running the show. Let me illustrate.

> Kayleah grew up in an abusive home. She was physically abused and neglected, but for her, the worst thing was the endless criticism. She worked hard to finish school with honors and go to college. School was an enjoyable challenge for her because she experienced success there. However, only a few months into an internship, Kayleah was feeling more stressed than ever. Every time her boss gave her a directive, it felt like a slap. Kayleah knew she needed help.
>
> At her first meeting with a counselor, Kayleah shared she had a "normal" childhood, but she struggled with criticism at work. During the session, she expressed herself as if she had no choices and was helpless.

Children are biologically wired to bond with their caregivers. Research has shown how incredibly important this is (Zeanah, 2005). When a young child is abused, be it physically, mentally, emotionally, socially, spiritually, sexually, or any combination of these, they will often still have a drive to bond with the abuser. They have very little recourse unless another safe adult can help them. Most children in a situation like this will develop the cognitive distortion of personalization. *Personalization* occurs when the child puts themselves at the center of everything wrong. This gives them power and some sense of control. After all, if they are the bad one, then they can just work on themselves to be better, and all will be well.

This usually does not work because the fault lies with the adult or environment, not the child. However, as no one can see what is happening inside another person's head, no one knows this is going on, and it becomes a hardwired way of engaging the world. Over time, erroneous beliefs cause the person to act out. This fortifies their belief in their "wrongness." Therefore, the adult facing an experience similar to the criticism of their childhood will react out of their younger self with all the feelings of helplessness. It takes the adult mind to come in and change the experience of the child brain.

Inner-child work is beyond what we can discuss here. Suffice it to say, Eye Movement Desensitization and Reprocessing (EMDR), Lifespan Integration (LI), guided imagery, narrative therapy, and internal family systems all provide different approaches to this valuable work. The important understanding for our discussion is to know that incidents and encounters from childhood often run the grown-up ship. Bringing the little one from the deep recesses of the brain into the present moment so they can share resources with the adult mind can be very healing.

However, when you first meet with someone and hear their litany of issues, it can be difficult to notice the child because they may sound sophisticated. In the adult, the child is often seen best through moods, behaviors, and physical reactions rather than thoughts and words. This brings us to two important types of memory: explicit and implicit memory. Just like that, we're back to having two systems to balance!

Dr. Jekyll and Mr. Hide—Semantic and Somatic Memory

Yes, I spelled it right . . . Mr. Hide. You will understand shortly.

The first type of memory system, our Dr. Jekyll—thought of as smart and wordy—is *explicit memory*, or declarative memory. This is memory tagged and filed in the brain via language. It is *semantic* and *episodic*, meaning the memory can be conveyed with words and relies on contextual cues and experience for filing and recall. There is a sense of time inherent with explicit memory. Autobiographical memory is a type of explicit memory.

Both the right and left brain are involved with explicit memory. To test this, go find someone, pick a day one to three days back, and ask them what they had for dinner. If you watch their face, you will notice most of them, while attempting to recall the memory, shift their eyes toward the right, and then quickly to the left, and then back to center. This is because they look to their right brain to see the picture of the food, go back to the left brain to retrieve the name of the food, and then look back at you to answer. Fascinating, isn't it?

The explicit system is also the type of memory most often accessed in talk-based therapy. Most of the challenges therapy clients face are not from issues in the explicit system, and therefore, they need experiential work in order to heal.

This brings us to out Mr. Hide, otherwise known as implicit memory (or procedural memory). *Implicit memory* is primarily emotional and sensory-based and is not time-tagged. It is deep, automatic memory. Try teaching a small child to tie their shoes or a teenager to drive a car, and you will run into challenges of implicit memory. This may be the type of memory most trouble-some in trauma as flashbacks. As associations can be made from just about anything, the person may not be aware of the reason for these frightening experiences. They can seem random and yet feel as if they are happening in the now. For therapists who treat trauma, it may be helpful to think of flashbacks and body memories as if they are happening again in the present moment.

Filing and Refiling the Files

As life is experienced, memories are consolidated. ***Consolidation*** occurs when memory is formed and filed the brain. In other words, it is what happens in the brain when neural pathways form a trace (or neural pathway) to a memory once it is stabilized (filed). Memory consolidation is crucial for a sense of coherence and well-being.

Consolidation may best occur when experiences are repeated and/or during sleep. It requires strong connections in the brain, and as you can imagine, the process of consolidation can be interrupted. How well, after all, are anxious, depressed, and traumatized people sleeping? With all the potential obstacles to consolidation, it is a relatively common occurrence to have retrieval errors due to cognitive distortions or inaccurate emotional tagging. For example, if your birthday cake fell, you may remember the whole birthday as terrible or feel an actual knot in your stomach every time you hear the words "birthday cake."

Explicit memory consolidation does not begin to occur in humans until around twelve to eighteen months of life. Whatever is consolidated is not particularly useful until around three to five years of age. Implicit memory, however, begins to form at birth (or even before, some say). A lot can happen before the age of three or four. This is why many people who come to treatment feel bad but have no idea why. It may also be the reason behind incongruent stories or behaviors.

There is good news though! If the process of consolidation is interrupted or something is misfiled or tagged with strong emotion or trauma, it can be reconsolidated. ***Reconsolidation*** is what happens when a memory is recalled and then re-stored. As mentioned above, this is a chief goal in treatment.

To understand this more fully, sit quietly (if you can) and close your eyes (after you read this next sentence). Try to recall a mildly unpleasant memory (open your eyes when you have a visual image). Now, on a piece of paper, write down a few things you can remember from that occasion. How do you feel? Now . . . imagine a kind and caring person asks about the event. Write down any memories or sensations you would experience then. Imagine further that the kind person encourages you often as you speak. Keep writing.

When finished, look at your list. Was there any difference in what you remembered, how you remembered it, or what you felt remembering it on your own versus imagining a caring friend?

Memory storage is labile. The very act of conjuring up a memory changes it, as does filing it after input. The more control, love, kindness, compassion, and other positive actions and emotions you experience during this process, the better you will feel about the memory. This makes reconsolidation an incredibly important therapeutic tool.

Memory Systems: Out of Balance?

Throughout this and the last section, I have stressed the importance of balance. It is no different with memory. People need to experience a balanced approach to working with the two types of memory: explicit and implicit.

As most of us are well-versed in dealing with semantic-based memory, a balanced approach will include elements for focus on implicit, somatic-based memory. The ideas shared above in the section "Right & Left Hemispheres: Out of Balance" may be useful here as well. Rather than talking here about the techniques to use, I want to address a particular mindset.

Throughout my years of counseling, I have had the honor of working with people who have what we call in the profession "personality disorders." I pray I live long enough to see a change in the name of this disorder. I realize the name implies the impact on the core of the person, but can you think of anything more unfortunate than being labeled with a disordered personality?

I am in the camp of those who believe we can take the personality disorders in general and break them into two categories. Category one would have philias, antisocials, psychopaths, and some narcissists. Category two would consist of borderline, histrionic, avoidant, and obsessive-compulsive personality disorders. For the first group, some now believe something with the mirror neuron system may be amiss. Perhaps there is faulty wiring or an absence of the ability to feel empathy (Fecteau, 2008). For the second cluster, though, the belief is that their issues stem from trauma, and the problem, so to speak, lies in the implicit memory.

As mentioned earlier, a great deal can happen before the age of three or four. Not only that, but trauma can also imprint directly onto the implicit memory in some cases. What this all means is the person with a personality disorder knows and feels something is wrong but is at war within between the *knowing* and *noetic* halves. Everything in their biology drives them to connect with life, others, and purpose. However, everything in their brain and all the memories in their body urge them to retreat. The push-pull trait of these disorders makes sense in this line of reasoning and does not stem from a flawed character.

This is all in its infancy, but I have seen the understanding of this work wonders with clients. Carrying a label indicating their very being is disordered causes these folks to be heavily defended and guarded. If approached as if they and their behaviors are defective, they will understandably recoil and resist. However, if we treat them as if they have memory issues, resistance from shame can be greatly reduced. When I meet someone with one of these diagnoses (or I suspect one of them), I tell them it is most likely a trauma response and our job is to reconsolidate healthier memory. Once they understand what this means, many people have cathartic releases. They still struggle greatly with their behavior, but they feel understood, acceptable, not so broken, and more willing to consider treatment recommendations.

"But wait!" you say. "Isn't your explanation and approach too simple?"

There is no doubt implicit memory issues wreak havoc on the brain, body, mind, and social aspects of life. Nothing is spared. However, it *is* simple. It is just not easy. This type of disorder runs deep and requires, most often, lengthy and intensive therapeutic work. This is why Dialectical Behavioral Therapy (DBT) is such a powerful and wonderful asset in the toolbox of not only those with so-called personality disorders, but anyone dealing with disorders of emotion regulation.

While we are building rapport, educating, and working to explore and repair memory, those we work with need to know how to manage their bodies and lives. Reducing the shame of the label may go a long way, but most still need to make up for years of shortfalls and discrepancies in social-emotional learning. For this, DBT is the gold standard of care, and I highly recommend that everyone struggling with any of the disorders mentioned today join a DBT group or seek treatment from a therapist who utilizes DBT treatment modalities.

You now know that to "right the ship" (bring healing and give hope) it is necessary to take a balanced therapeutic approach for several body systems. We now return our focus to anxiety and continue the trend of duos as we look at the two paths to anxiety.

Tips & Tricks (For the Journey of Recovery)

As a caregiver, especially in the beginning, it is not necessary to dig too deeply into memory. Remember the BFFs—the hippocampus and amygdala? It's more important to drill into emotions attached to the memories. These often tell more of the story than our words. To become more aware and observant of emotional underpinnings, try one of these exercises:

1. Go to the mall or a coffee shop and watch people talking. Try to guess their emotional state.
2. Find an emotional television show or movie. Play it without the volume on and see if you can guess what they are feeling.
3. Ask a friend or family member to tell you about a memory. Ask clarifying questions based solely on the emotion you are noticing or is lacking.

Chapter Challenge Questions (Cortex Focus)

1. What does it mean to you to know memory is for the future?
2. How did you do with the test? What did you learn? How does it change your perspective on memory?
3. How much time do you spend drilling people for their memories? Do you count them as facts? How does this affect your relationships?
4. Journal about the difference between explicit and implicit memory and how knowing about them will affect you.

Go Deeper (Somatic Focus)

1. **Narrative therapy** is an incredibly useful technique, as it allows the brain to make sense of life. Consider writing a timeline. It does not have to span your entire life. Start and

end somewhere. Over days or weeks, spend a few minutes every day visualizing, pondering over, and maybe even asking others about the time. Write about what you learn. Add to your timeline. Did you discover anything along the way?

2. **Mindfulness**. Find a quiet location and give yourself fifteen minutes of uninterrupted time to attempt this exercise. Take a deep breath and close your eyes (after you read this, of course). Notice the smells, sounds, sights, tastes, and sensations through your skin. Then look around the room. Ground yourself in the present moment. As you relax, allow thoughts and memories to come into your awareness. When one piques your interest, allow your mind to linger. Notice all the sensations, thoughts, and actions you can for approximately five minutes. Then, move on to a different meditation. Examples: Count your breaths. Take a mindfulness walk. Do some mindful dishwashing. Leave the memory for at least five minutes. Then, return and allow the memory to come into your awareness again. Notice any differences. Journal about your experience.

CHAPTER SIX

The Two Paths

AREN'T OUR BODIES amazing? Two sides of the brain, two regulatory systems, two processing systems, and two memory systems to be addressed in a balanced manner. Remember, balance does not always mean equal. Knowing when these are out of balance or not working well together (integrated) are important guideposts in therapy.

Now for another twofer: two paths to anxiety—neural paths, that is. Knowing the difference is the key to choosing informed treatment.

The Great Confusion

In technical terms, the two pathways are called the "amygdala path" and the "cortex path." With the amygdala path, anxiety is caused by somatic triggers. In the cortex path, however, anxiety is instigated by thoughts. However, as you learned earlier, the amygdala/limbic system is responsible for the somatic sensations of anxiety in the body. No amygdala, no feeling of anxiety. Therefore, in all cases, the amygdala is activated.

Confused? I know. I was too.

To make things clearer, I will use different terms to refer to these two pathways. When anxiety is ignited by thinking (or other processes in the cortex), I will use the term "top-down anxiety." However, when anxiety occurs in the body without a thought-based trigger, it will be referred to as "bottom-up anxiety."

Top-Down and Bottom-Up Anxiety

Top-down anxiety occurs when thoughts originating in the cortex signal alarm to the amygdala. For example, imagine yourself walking home from the park on a sunny summer day, without a care in the world. In the distance, you hear the siren of a fire engine. Initially, this is of no concern. You hear fire engines all the time. However, as the sound grows louder and nearer, your brain suggests, "Oh no! What if it's my house on fire?" Instantly, the amygdala springs into action, and your meandering walk morphs into a sprint for home. Finding your home just fine, the amygdala relaxes, and all is well. You realize your thought was in error and likely understand that the anxiety came from the thinking. Once the stand-down message is sent, balance is restored (though you're likely to embellish the story some when you retell it later).

With **bottom-up anxiety**, the trigger may not be easily discerned in the present moment. Suppose as a child, your bedroom was painted an unusual hue of teal. Now, imagine each time you went into your room, your brother punched you in the arm and took your toys. Over time, your brain may associate the color of the room with danger. The amygdala, being a cautious "over-generalizer," tends to play it safe. This means any time the brain registers the color teal, the amygdala goes on alert. Twenty years later and hundreds of miles away, the color teal may make you feel uneasy for no reason you can point to in the present moment—even if your brother is your best friend now. This is an example of bottom-up, somatic-influenced anxiety.

Our Friend, the Thalamus

Let's look a little closer at how this works. Consider the diagram below.

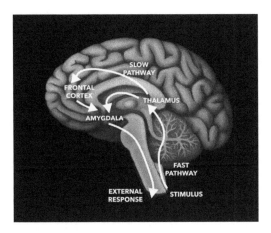

Magic is happening in this picture.

Remember our friend the thalamus, a.k.a. "Grand Central Station"? When a stimulus is perceived by our sensory organs, the information passes through the thalamus. When something has been tagged as a known danger, the thalamus routes the information directly to the amygdala along what's called the *fast path*. If, however, more information is needed to determine a threat, then the amygdala stays quiet as the information travels the *slow path* through the cortex first.

Take a minute to imagine the implications of this. Can you think of examples of the two paths?

Glitches in the System

While you ponder, let me warn you there can be problems along the way. Besides sensory errors, not everything tagged as a known threat is actually a threat.

What? You mean I could be afraid but there might not be any threat?

Yes. That is what I mean.

To start, humans are born with only two fears: falling and loud noises.

You might say, "Wait a minute! Aren't we afraid of dying?"

Have you seen a two-year-old climb up things? We are not afraid of dying.

"Well," you continue, "what about starving? Surely we're afraid of starving!"

Babies cry *expecting* their parents to come to feed and care for them. No, we are not born afraid of starving. We only become so if we experience it after birth.

"Okay," you say, "surely we social creatures are afraid of abandonment. Certainly *that* is feared from birth."

Again, no. As with hunger, babies have cries to indicate the need for human contact. We are born anticipating and expecting love, safety, and connection. Only when these are absent do fears emerge.

Babies come into the world dependent and initially function using their right brain, somatic experiencing, and implicit memory. For a small child, *any* threats to safety and well-being is a threat to life and limb. Criticism, for example, may result in loss of love, food, or privileges. A child who experiences enough of these issues can develop anxiety or other mental health issues. If it is bad enough, they may have failure to thrive, other medical issues, or even death.

Fears can develop in a child and work well when they are small, but not so well as they reach adulthood. This is what I mean when I say not all threats are real. If the threat no longer exists but the triggers do, then interpretive errors occur along the two paths. The job of the therapist, then, is to help the client identify and learn to react differently to these glitches. To do this practically, let us look at one more possible way-of-thinking delineation: fear vs. anxiety.

Fear vs. Anxiety

If the body feels racked with unpleasant sensations and the brain is twirling a million miles a minute, how is a person to have any idea which path is being activated? One way is to teach them a sort of threat analysis.

What is the purpose of the fast path? Why does the thalamus bypass the cortex when there is danger? In essence, to keep us safe and alive. Safe from what, then? Primarily, safe from threats to life and limb—such as falling debris, fire, and other natural disasters—and physical harm from animals and others. This response I will name *fear*.

However, not every danger we encounter is a threat to our very life and physical well-being. The majority of perils most people face in the modern Western world are more along the lines of threats to social standing. These may include disappointing others, facing criticism or rejection, or somehow losing position, power, and status with loved ones or in the community. In addition to this, there is the potential to perceive a non-actual threat to life and limb. Examples of this would be the feelings produced by OCD (such as fearing you will die if you don't tap the doorknob), reacting in the present to a danger from the past, or believing you will face harm or death with no current evidence to support it. All these types of threats I will call *anxiety*.

Jimmy Moves to Istanbul

Read the following story and see if you can tease out what is anxiety versus fear.

> Jimmy could hardly stand still, he was so excited! The day had finally come. He had waited three long years for the promotion and relocation. He could hardly believe he was going to move to Istanbul! Being of Turkish

descent, he had long had a fascination with the country, the only one in the world in both Asia and Europe! Though he had never been before, he felt he was going home.

The phone rang, jolting Jimmy out of his daydream. The Uber had arrived. Not wanting to keep the driver waiting, he grabbed his bags, took one last look at his apartment, and hurried out the door. Five minutes into the ride, panic began to overtake him as he realized he had left his phone at home. In a tone uncharacteristic of his usually mild manner, Jimmy shouted at the Uber driver to turn around. Dutifully, albeit with irritation, the driver complied. Jimmy, heart racing, face flushed, and stomach churning, returned to his flat and retrieved his phone.

Upon his return to the car, things really became dodgy. They finally arrived at the airport, forty-five minutes late. Familiar feelings of dread overtook him, initiating the start of an internal war. Feeling bad at his earlier treatment of the driver, yet in a hurry, Jimmy halfheartedly apologized as he pushed the buttons on his phone and jumped out of the back seat. He grabbed his bag and ran into the terminal.

Standing in the check-your-bag line, his thoughts felt as if they were swirling, one bumping into the other. He realized he had forgotten to tip the driver. This awareness only served to further agitate him. *Oh man!* he thought, *I can't even get to the airport without problems! How on earth will I handle living in a foreign country and managing a team? I'll surely be fired, and then I will have to come back and live in a hole.*

The lady behind the check-in counter called "Next" three times before Jimmy finally heard her. Once relieved of his bag, Jimmy found his gate with fifteen minutes to spare! He was amazed. Hungry, yet still battling negative thinking, Jimmy thought he would surely choke if he tried to eat anything. The flight would be long, though, and he was not a fan of airplane food. His growling stomach eventually won, and he made his way to the Hudson shop to find some food.

The airport was exceptionally crowded. Jimmy found himself leaping out of the way of golf carts and dogs on leashes. Ten minutes later, armed with a Mexi-melt bagel and a can of Sprite, he arrived back at the gate just in time to board. Doubt had found room in his mind, but at least he was on the plane.

Ever experience anything like this? What did you notice? Did you see the top-down and bottom-up pathways firing or notice the instances of fear as opposed to anxiety? The proportions used in this story are intended to mirror what one might experience in life, meaning there are far more instances of anxiety than fear. Let's analyze this and see what we find.

Threat Analysis

What are some of the threats you noticed in the story? Here is the list I propose. Try to guess which type of threat each of these is: fear or anxiety?

Point to Analyze
Panic overtaking him as he realized he lost his phone
Heart racing when he ran to get his phone
Feelings of dread about missing the plane (45 minutes late)
Agitated at not leaving a tip
Certain he would choke on his food
He leaped out of the way of oncoming traffic

What type of threats are these?

Point to Analyze	Threat Type
Panic at losing his phone	Anxiety—Threat to Social Standing (if he loses his phone, he may have to inconvenience others as he figures things out without it) OR Non-Actual Threat to Life and Limb (assuming he cannot live without the phone)
Heart racing as he runs to his apartment to retrieve the phone	Anxiety—Threat to Social Standing (does not want to be late to the airport, miss the plane, and cause inconvenience)
Dread of being late to the airport	Anxiety—Same reason as above
Agitated at not leaving a tip for the driver	Anxiety—Threat to Social Standing (fear of being thought of in a negative light)
He feared he would choke on his food	Anxiety—Non-Actual Threat to Life & Limb (was not choking in the present moment and was more concerned about making a spectacle of himself than actually choking)
Leaping out of the way of oncoming traffic	Fear—Threat to Life & Limb (being hit by a car is an actual danger)

Wow! Really? There was only one thing to fear in all of Jimmy's story?

Yes, just one. Only the potential of being run over by the airport shuttle would harm him.

Now, think about your life and your daily troubles. Map out your day like Jimmy's. How much of what you deal with is an *actual* threat to life and limb?

Why am I being so persnickety about separating fear and anxiety? I'll answer you with a question: What is the appropriate response to fear (threats to life and limb)? Do you hear Jeopardy music in the background? Why, yes, Alex, the answer is "What is fight or flight?" Whenever our well-being is at stake, we need to get help or get out. Have you noticed, though, that since the amygdala fires in both scenarios, many people who are not under actual threat of imminent harm still react with fight or flight? Their method may be more subtle. They may be chronically angry or frustrated, or they might avoid connection altogether. These responses do not help fortify our position in the social world, do they?

Here's another question, then: What is the appropriate response to anxiety (threats to social standing or non-actual threats to life and limb)?

Rest and think a minute here before you read the answer. Once a person realizes they are safe, pretty much all they need to do is learn the appropriate response to these types of threats.

"What's are the appropriate responses?" you ask with bated breath.

Problem solving, people skills, and distress tolerance. These are the appropriate responses to anxiety.

To bring it all together for you, here's another lovely chart:

FEAR	ANXIETY
Represents Threats to: LIFE & LIMB	Represents Threats to: Social Standing & Non-Actual Threats/Dangers
Fast-Path Response in the Brain; Limbic/Motor Response Takes over Body Functions	Slow-path Response in the Brain; Mindfulness Awareness Required
Appropriate Response to Fear: Fight or Flight	Appropriate Response to Anxiety: People Skills Problem Solving Distress Tolerance

Seeing clearly which type of threat you or others are facing can help reduce unhelpful responses to anxiety as you realize you are, in fact, going to live to fight another day.

The Two Paths in a Nutshell

Amygdala—"Bottom-Up"—Path	Cortex—"Top-Down"—Path
Bottom-Up	Top-Down
Primarily Somatic; may not have an understanding as to the cause of anxiety	Primarily triggered by thinking; root of anxiety may be more easily known
Primarily Fast Path	Primarily Slow Path
Fear: Threats to Life and Limb	Anxiety: Threats to Social Standing
Example: Ducking when a baseball is flying at your head	Example: Thinking you better call 911 when you hear someone trying to open your front door at 2 a.m.

Amygdala—"Bottom-Up"—Path	Cortex—"Top-Down"—Path
Proper Response: Fight or Flight	Proper Response: People Skills, Problem Solving, Distress Tolerance
Glitch Response: Jumping out of the way of a "snake" that is actually a sock	Glitch Response: Justifying your partner after they have hit you
Proper Response: Calm the Body and Mind	Proper Response: Cultivate Accurate/Constructive Cognitive Practices

Tips & Tricks (For the Journey of Recovery)

One of the most crucial lessons we can learn in the recovery journey is to slow down! This is far easier said than done, as people around us will add pressure to move us along. Learning to manage the anxiety from waiting and giving yourself permission to allow others to do the same can be freeing. Here are some ideas for practice.

- Spend a day counting slowly to three or four before you respond to anyone who talks to you.
- Close your eyes and try to visualize what has happened or what might happen before you take any action.
- Think about the last two or three times you had unpleasant interactions or something went wrong for you. Was fast-path responding involved? Write down what you would do differently should the same situation occur again.

Chapter Challenge Questions (Cortex Focus)

1. Can you recall instances in your own life when you experienced fast-path and slow-path anxiety? Were they accurate?
2. Think about the last time you were upset with someone

you care about. How does knowing we all have fast- and slow-path responses affect your thoughts about the given situation?

3.   Write out a plan for catching yourself in an erroneous fast-path response.

Go Deeper (Somatic Focus)

Expressive Art. Find a large piece of construction paper and fold it into four quarters. Open it so that you see one sheet with four squares. In square one, draw yourself in an appropriate fast-path response. In square two, draw yourself in an appropriate slow-path response. In square three, draw yourself in an erroneous fast-path response (when you acted fast but would have done better to slow down). In square four, draw yourself in an erroneous slow-path response (when you overanalyzed and would have done better to act quickly). Look at the picture. Put it away for a few days. Open it again and then journal your reaction.

Mindfulness Activity. Learn the Breath Sabbath (Muller, 2000). For this, think of something you do regularly each day—like walk through a particular door or make a meal—or choose a time you can regularly remember throughout the day, such as the top of the hour. Now, think of a favorite quote, scripture, or saying that inspires you. Maybe it will be a picture and not words. Every time you do the preselected thing each day, stop, take a deep, cleansing breath, and say your words or envision your picture in your mind. Then whisper some gratitude for the momentary break.

CHAPTER SEVEN

Teaching Neuroscience to Others: Analogies and Simplifications

Ready, Set, Teach!

WHAT A RIDE! You have added many new ideas to your recovery toolbox. Now it is time to teach it to someone else. They say the best way to learn is to teach. You ready?

In case the idea seems daunting to you, I will give you an example of how I go about it. Everyone will be different. You are a magnificent and creative creature. (Tap into your right brain, you analytical types! It's all in there.) You can take my examples, elaborate on them, and make them your own. It may be helpful to think from a learner's perspective as you read. Here goes!

But I Want to Ride the Bicycle Too!

As you learned in the study of memory, the brain is an anticipation engine. If a person has no idea what someone else wants them to do, it will be very difficult for them to fully participate. Being a warm and fuzzy type is not enough for others to grab onto for trust.

Think of it this way: Imagine someone you know said, "Let's go on a trip," and he gave you no further information—what would you think? If, however, he said, "Let's go on a trip to New York. It will take seven days, and we will take my truck. We will stop any time we need to and spend each night in a hotel." You still do not know everything, but you know some important parameters. Even if you had a strong relationship with the person suggesting the trip, you would probably appreciate (to say the least) the second option more than the first.

We therapists essentially say to our clients, "Come, let's go on a trip. It will be painful, but I'll be right there with you." Nice as the sentiment is, can you see a problem? The person on the receiving end will struggle to understand the journey and will naturally, and often nonconsciously, resist.

Therefore, one of the first things I do is explain that therapy is about exploring and learning, and I want them to know how learning happens. *Learning* is the process by which experience and knowledge are acquired and integrated, and it occurs with the help of all areas of the brain. It requires the entire body as well as the environment. Yes, the whole kit and kaboodle!

Imagine you were two years old and you had never seen a bicycle before. This is where learning begins—at the point where we do not know what we do not know. This level of learning is called *unconscious-unskilled*. We are generally pretty content at this level. Here, for example, we would have no idea bicycles exist and therefore do not care that we cannot ride one.

Suppose, however, a time comes when we see another child down the block riding a bike. It looks like fun, and we decide we want to learn to do it too. This state of being is called *conscious-unskilled*. People tend to be uncomfortable in this stage. We struggle with not knowing how to do something we want to do. This may be particularly difficult if we assume that simply knowing about something means we should know how to do it—a virtual mischief-maker in recovery.

Eventually, though, we jump on the bike and practice and learn to ride it. That is all well and good, but we must use a great deal of conscious energy, as we must think through every step over and over. It is tiring, and we may complain, "It doesn't feel natural." We also may have many wipeouts. This level of learning is called ***conscious-skilled***. We tend to not like this level of learning at all. We always want to look like pros at everything. Therefore, this is where most people would quit if not encouraged in some way.

With consistent practice (the duration of which depends on many factors), we one day jump on the bike, and off we go— no highly conscious thought involved any longer. This final stage is called ***unconscious-skilled*** (also known as automatic). Here is where we spend most of our lives, and it is the place where we are happiest. Well, until we're not.

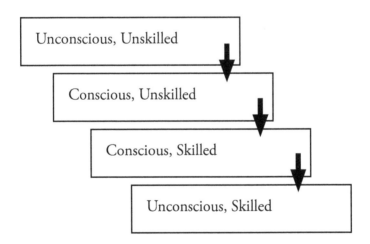

Sometimes, we discover something is no longer effective for us. For example, if a parent was covert in how they spoke with us, and questions were disguises for digs and insults (such as "Don't you want the light on, Sweetie?" as code for "Get up, lazy! Can't you turn the light on by yourself?"), we could hear all questions as accusations and may snap at anyone who asks something.

If we realize some of what we have learned was in error or no longer working for us, would we have to start all over at unconscious-unskilled? No, we already have awareness. We may spend some time on the second level, learning some new skills—but mostly, we will have to use what we have learned in a very conscious, careful manner to become more proficient at proper use.

Therefore, my job as a therapist and teacher, often, is to take the listener back to conscious-skilled, which can be uncomfortable. Helping people see therapy as a learning process whose goal is to eventually return to unconscious-skilled, or automatic, may make it easier for them. This can provide some landmarks for the journey and relieve some distress along the way.

Ways to Think about Brain Science

Whew! Still with me? You're doing great! It is not necessary to try to explain everything you have learned. You need to understand the underlying processes to know when to apply which concept. Most people need to have enough to satisfy the "anticipation engine." This could vary from person to person.

The Brain. Dr. Dan Siegel uses a simple "hand model" of the brain (Siegel, 2010). This refers to the triune brain (from chapter three, "Therapeutic Neuroscience"), and refers to the "lizard brain" (brain stem and cerebellum), the "emotional brain" (amygdala area), and the "the thinking brain" (frontal, temporal, and parietal lobes). This language is not always clear or acceptable to all people. You may need to experiment to figure out the best wording to use.

What follows is a script I created, and you can use it to explain the brain to others. Extra information for inquisitive minds may need to come from the reference list at the end of this book. Be encouraged to make adaptations to this to fit your understanding and personality. It will be best if conveyed authentically (or you may use this transcript as a reading assignment, with due credit included).

(First, explain about the whole person, you are not your brain, and learning.)

When thinking about the brain, it can be helpful to think in terms of roles rather than structures. For example, the frontal lobe houses what is known as ***executive function***. This area we will call the *executive assistant* (EA)—the guidance system in charge of "driving the ship" when left on autopilot.

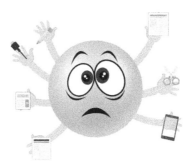

The EA does many things at once but is limited to a maximum of seven internal and/or external processes (such as processing cold skin, thoughts of anger, bright lights, a stomachache, and someone shouting your name). This process utilizes ***working memory***. When working memory is overloaded or impaired, you may feel easily overwhelmed and unable to think clearly. This is common in many mental health disorders.

The File Cabinet. The rest of the brain beyond the prefrontal cortex can be thought of as a file cabinet. This part houses all the rules for safety and efficiency. There are both conscious and nonconscious files. Therefore, the file cabinet includes experiences, perceptions, and memories. The neural networks connect the EA to the file cabinet and can be described as "couriers" (or for children, as "minions"). Couriers/minions use a map of neural pathways to find files.

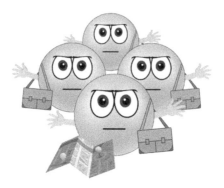

As you know, you breathe without any conscious effort, though you can hold your breath or speed up/slow down your breathing at will. Accessing the files is similar. It can happen in two different ways: manually or automatically. A memory can pop into your mind, as if the couriers/minions retrieved the files on their own, through a trigger of some sort (though we are not always aware of it). Or the EA can search for a memory. Automatic memory recall is often tremendously faster than conscious recall.

When memories are triggered by nonconscious, pre-existing vulnerability factors, it can cause some issues. Imagine you grew up with a sibling who did not value your time. They were always late, with no remorse or apology. This left you feeling uncared for and angry. Flash forward a few years. You are waiting at a restaurant for your friend, who turns out to be ten minutes late. You want to scream! It's a minor infraction in the scheme of things, but because you were not consciously aware of how your past experience relates to what is happening in the present, the couriers have been triggered and have run off to the "blow-your-top" file.

With some training, the EA can learn to pay attention to or ignore certain stimuli. In the situation with the late friend, once the vulnerability factor has been identified, the EA will realize this present moment is different from times with the sibling. The courier, then, will be sent to retrieve the "concern" file or the "draw-a-new-boundary" file. In this case, no strong emotional files are needed, and the system stays in balance (there's that word again!).

There are other important qualities of the files to note, namely: you may not be the main filer, the files cannot be replaced easily, they are not always accurate, and they can be changed or misplaced.

Who Files the Files? It may be surprising (and disconcerting) to realize you may not be the main one in charge of choosing what is added to the file cabinet. What do I mean? There are many ways to create a file.

> ➢ Sheer repetition. If you hear something often enough, you might come to believe it.
> ➢ Borrowing it. Otherwise known as taking it on authority. This means you believe the person who told you.
> ➢ Liking it. If you like what you hear, it goes in the file.
> ➢ The file's importance. If it matters to you, you'll record it.

We do not often analyze what is in our file system. It is possible to be unaware of a belief you hold until you notice the actions, words, or thoughts generated by the belief. It is always best if we can choose the files we need mindfully. However, no one is aware of what they are doing every minute. Therefore, it is helpful to find a way to remember the influence the files have on us when we are in autopilot and to create checkpoints or cues to help us self-correct. Sticky notes, routines, and accountability partners are all ways to do this.

Replacing a File. Have you ever had an "ah-ha! moment" regarding a needed change, only to return to your old behavior? Simply raising awareness is not enough to integrate changes into the efficient autopilot system. This is a safety issue. Let's say you read a manual that explains how to fly a plane. Having never done it before, you have no muscle memory, nor have you learned any related emotional cues. Imagine you sign up for a lesson but tell your teacher you do not need to be told how to land because you already know. Suffice it to say, you would not be around long if your thought patterns and emotional states changed quickly in such a case. It is important for the file cabinet to contain only tried and trusted files. Summation: emotions do not change first or fast.

Even so, not all the files are accurate, even those you have had a long time. Just because you feel a certain way or think something is true, does not make it so. For example, just because your dad calls you lazy does not make it true. You need patience, wisdom, and experience to sort through the files and weed out errors. Then you need perseverance to replace them with the truth.

Changing and Misplacing Files. An example of a changed file is when you recall your birthday and remember your friend Joe there—and he says he didn't go that year. A misplaced file is when you forget something.

Meet SAM. As you have learned, the EA is the flexible, in-the-moment part of you. It gathers information that you can use to make decisions and to understand your world. Your brain is very complex, and the aware part is not the only part at work at any time. You also have another significant player we'll call "SAM."

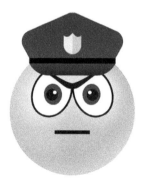

SAM is an acronym first coined by Dr. Dan Siegel, and it stands for *search*, *alert*, and *mobilize* (Siegel, 2010). SAM's job is to keep you safe from physical danger. SAM lives in the emotional part of your brain, relatively close to the survival area. Think of SAM as the fight-or-flight system. SAM can hear the EA and understand warnings. However, the connections to the EA do not always go both ways. By this, I mean, the EA (and you) may not always know why SAM is on the alert.

There are some more helpful things to know about SAM. First, SAM is extraordinarily fast in comparison to the EA. Think of SAM as the Cray supercomputer and the EA as the first IBM computer. Yup . . . before dial-up! This means SAM is often aware of danger and begins to ring the warning bell (which is felt as fear or anxiety in your body) and push you out of the way (via your motor cortex) before the EA even knows what has happened. In other words, anxiety and other upsetting emotions can be triggered by something only SAM can see. The trigger is often something hurtful from the past and is noticed physically through your senses (such as seeing a familiar pattern of behavior, smelling a particular food, or hearing a door slam). You may not be aware of the trigger. You may just feel bad.

Nevertheless, SAM does not always act first. Sometimes, SAM is minding his own business, thinking everything is going fine, when the EA says something scary. Imagine you're sitting comfortably at home in your living room when you hear the garage door open. The door opening on its own does not incite any reaction from SAM. However, if the EA suddenly says, "Who's opening the garage? I'm the only one home today!" then this could greatly upset SAM. Therefore, sometimes your thoughts ignite anxiety and upset—and these thoughts are also not always accurate. This is the reason a therapist or other care provider will focus on both helping you change the way you think *and* helping you learn to calm your anxious body (when the source of the fear is not accurate or not truly present).

The Family in Your Brain

We are all "someone else" from time to time. Ever known someone who was the life of the party until they walked into the door of their parents' house? Suddenly, they are quiet and demure. You may feel as if the body snatchers have returned.

As we grow and learn, we develop patterns of behavior that are situational and environment specific. Because of this and how the brain itself works, it can be helpful to think of different areas of your brain as family members. These family members want to watch after you, and they are in charge of various areas of the file systems. They are highly rule driven and emotional. Consider the following picture:

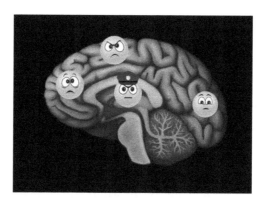

In the frontal lobe of the brain, where executive functioning, organization, and planning take place is the Worrier (who may sometimes act as the EA). This character is in the present moment and aware of consequences and the future. Obviously, the Worrier worries.

Next, a bit farther back in the brain (in or near the insulate), we have the Bully. This part of the brain may have some current-moment awareness but may be trigger-based. The Bully might antagonize you or others. The goal is to keep you in line or in power, in the status quo, or following rules developed to keep you safe. The Bully is forceful because of the perceived consequences if you do not behave the way the Bully wants.

We met SAM. SAM resides in the lower, central part of the brain. SAM can be thought of as the amygdala or limbic system. When SAM is active, the body feels sensations and may engage in anxiety behaviors. SAM makes the body uncomfortable. SAM is not in the current moment and is purely trigger-based.

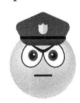

Finally, far back in the deepest part of the brain is the Child. The Child is also highly emotional and somatic. The Child could engage with the Worrier, the Bully, or SAM. How you know a Child is running the show is the feeling of being small, helpless, or abandoned.

The important thing to understand about the family members is none of them is you. You are the parent, boss, teacher, programmer, pilot—whatever word seems to fit. It is your job to listen to each member but not to be swayed by them if their distress is not accurate to the present moment. Remember, each of these parts of you was developed over time and may not always reflect the needs of the present. The goal is to improve your hearing of each one and to give direction and even override, as needed.

Note for those who use Internal Family Systems (IFS)—a therapy that presumes we all have different mental sides to ourselves: The Worrier and the Bully are Managers, and the Child is, of course, an Exile. SAM, depending on what is happening, could be a Firefighter.

Interacting with the Family

This concept has proven to be very helpful in separating the diagnoses of anxiety, depression, or trauma from the client. Remember: you are not your brain.

Many people dealing with troubling emotions have a difficult time separating themselves from the things they do and the experiences they have. One way to create health is to engage in compassionate and realistic self-talk. However, attempting to do this directly can be difficult. Therefore, engaging this concept as a way to slowly bring a person close to their wounded parts may be helpful.

I will share three family-in-the-brain assignments I often give.

- ✓ **Represent Them.** Once the parts-of-the-brain concept has been explained, I ask the person to take the week to imagine each of the parts and then show me what they come up with. I usually say, "Represent them for me." Give as little direction as possible. It has been fascinating to see what people see. I've seen parents, siblings, colors, fictional characters, and even songs.
- ✓ **Who's in Charge?** Once a mental image has been created for each, I ask my client to spend a week noticing who is running the show. I will often encourage them to add reminders on their phone to prompt them to check in and ask. I have yet to have someone not be able to answer this question. It is very helpful to learn whether the Worrier, the Bully, SAM, or the Child is heard from most.
- ✓ **How Do You Interact?** Once they are aware of who is in charge, have them spend time noticing how they respond. This is when you can introduce the idea of reframing and self-compassion. If the Bully is on a rampage, it is because they are worried. Instead of ignoring the Bully, yelling at

him to shut up, or agreeing, one might simply attempt to understand what he wants and state it consciously in a positive reframe. Example: Bully says, "You're such an idiot for missing that appointment!" This could be restated as, "The Bully sees I did not prepare for the meeting and is worried about the consequences." Have your client restate it to themselves the way they would want to hear it.

There are many right-brained, image-based ways to use this family. Asking "who is talking?" when you hear negative self-speak or having them practice talking to those parts may also be helpful.

Tips & Tricks (For the Journey of Recovery)

It is very easy to forget that people new to the healing journey (or who have worked with others in the past) may not know all the same things you do. You might feel frustrated when they move slowly or resist. Resistance often stems from four main areas:

1. The person does not understand the therapeutic process.
2. There is fear of the outcome.
3. The person has no frame of reference for what healthy living is.
4. The person's identity is wrapped up in the problem they say they want to solve.

Consider sitting down and writing out the names of people who frustrate you and see if you can guess which of the above four reasons they might have for their resistance. How can you help?

Chapter Challenge Questions (Cortex Focus)

1. How does knowing the levels of learning help a person better understand therapy?

2. How would you explain the brain to someone else? Try it out.

3. SAM does not act because we want SAM to act. SAM acts on triggers. What does his knowledge do for you? How would you explain this to others?

4. How will you use the family-in-the-brain concept?

Go Deeper (Somatic Focus)

Expressive Art. Represent the family in *your* brain. Journal about your reaction.

Visual Imagery. Sit down with your picture of the family in your brain and mentally visualize each one. Imagine how they look and what they sound like; maybe they even have a smell. Imagine yourself giving each one of them a hug. What would you thank them for? Is there any constructive criticism or requests you have for them? Deliver those with kindness and compassion. Journal about the experience.

PART II

Somatic & Cognitive Applications

CHAPTER EIGHT

The Fast Path: Dealing with Amygdala-Based Anxiety

"**W**OW! ARE WE finally getting to the nitty-gritty of how to deal with anxiety?" you ask. Why yes—yes, we are!

For those of you reading this book who are not therapists, counselors, or other professionals in the mental health field, please keep reading. What follows may have a clinical flavor, but the stories and examples will likely resonate with you, and you will therefore find validation. If the techniques sound promising, you will know what to ask for in treatment. Feel free to dig deep or just skim.

Let's jump in.

Slow the Heck Down!

Our world moves at a rapid pace, and therapy can as well. Suppose Maurice comes into therapy to deal with work-related stress. He wants to ask his boss for a raise, but his fear prevents him. He meets his therapist, and they commence work together. Over the first few weeks, they start on the foundation of therapy: building rapport. In doing this, the therapist asks Maurice a few opening questions. It may go something like this:

> **Therapist:** So nice to meet you, Maurice. (Therapist shares credentials and background.) What brings you in to see me?
>
> **Maurice:** Nice to meet you too. Well, I need to ask my boss for a raise. I'm a good worker and it's been long enough, but the guy just freaks me out. I just stammer and can't say anything when I'm with him. I have always had this problem, and I figured now that I have a kid on the way, I should work on it.
>
> **Therapist:** Wonderful! Sounds like learning to talk to the boss would enhance your life and reduce some stress as you prepare for the changes in your family.
>
> **Maurice:** Yes. I think so.
>
> **Therapist:** So tell me, Maurice . . . what strengths do you have to help you reach your goals?
>
> (Extended silence while Maurice looks like a deer in headlights.)
>
> **Maurice:** Umm . . . well. I don't know. I'm kind of awkward socially. I'm not sure I have any.
>
> **Therapist:** Surely you do! After all, you came here today, didn't you? That's a strength.
>
> **Maurice:** I guess so. *Doesn't feel like a strength to me. I feel like coming here means I'm defective and need fixing. Guess it takes a lot of strength to drag yourself to the therapist when everyone around you knows it's because you're a loser.*
>
> **Therapist:** Great. Let's create some goals!

I am being a bit silly here . . . this interaction would most certainly take longer and be more in-depth, but what is of note is the therapist missed the most foundational goal in anxiety therapy: identify your assets!

If someone with anxiety is unable to identify any strengths, then the first goal needs to be to go on a quest to find or obtain some. We often breeze right past this necessary step, probably for two main reasons. First, we struggle to meet them exactly where they are—which can feel pretty low—and the truth could very well be that for what they want to do, they don't have many related strengths. We do not know how to state this, which leads to simply assuming they will instantly adopt our belief system.

Do not feel bad about this. Everything in society and your training has set you up for this. Most of us are meant to meet a new client, build rapport, diagnose, and create goals within the first session or two—which is clinically impossible. Therefore, we need to think of this process as a living organism that starts with first impressions but grows over time.

Also, very few of us have ever had any training in pedagogy. Some of you reading this do not even know the word. *Pedagogy* is the science of teaching. Knowing something does not mean you can impart it to others. It is rather difficult to convert book learning to practical application. Without the knowledge and understanding of how to do this, we often fall into the very attractive pit of believing that simply telling a person what we know is the job. It is not.

Therefore, take time to notice and develop the strengths your client needs to accomplish the desired goal. Make it an assignment. Have them write down any strengths they notice, or others point out to them. If you give this as an assignment, do not forget to give them permission to have strengths. It is not arrogant, selfish, or overconfident to notice and remark on your own strengths and accomplishments.

Think about this too: If a person wants to buy a house, there is no point in meeting the real-estate agent until that person has savings and a strong enough credit rating. Likewise, let's not expect Maurice to talk to his boss if he is unable to gather his thoughts under pressure. It may be more helpful to practice what he is learning in the office by having mock conversations and role plays.

The foundation of therapeutic alliance, besides building rapport and ensuring the client is safe, is discovering, building, and validating their strengths.

Don't Skip Step One!

Once you have built rapport, educated your client on pertinent aspects of mind, body, and spirit, and taught them the prerequisite skills needed for the therapy you are about to do, you are finally ready to begin treatment. It is true. These steps must occur before you start. I would go so far as to say real therapy may not even begin until both the therapist and the client are in the present moment, sharing at least the beginnings of a common reality. One cannot change a story they do not yet own.

I digress.

Interestingly, in all my work in treating anxiety over the years, one trend that stands out strongest to me at this point is the non-sequitur approach of skipping the first step.

What do I mean?

Let's return to Maurice. He wants to ask his boss for a raise, right? I imagine the first few weeks of therapy would unfold as follows. After a session or two of getting to know him, the therapist would work to understand the contributors to Maurice's fear of the boss. Perhaps they would teach some relaxation skills and maybe even a CBT skill or two. The therapist may go so far as to prescribe a few instances of behavioral practice with lesser fears. After debriefing and processing all this, Maurice will be relaxed and comfortable in therapy and will appear to have made some progress.

> **Therapist:** I have noticed some real progress with you since we met! On the first day, you had difficulty making eye contact with me. Even gathering your thoughts seemed a chore at times. However, now you talk with ease, and you have really learned those cognitive distortions. Way to go! You seem more relaxed and confident as well! You think you're ready to go talk to your boss?
>
> **Maurice:** (borrowing the therapist's energy and confidence) Yes, I do! I mean, it has been so nice to open up and talk to you. I have been able to say things I usually couldn't. It feels good. I think after our weekly staff meeting on Thursday, I'll ask for a time to talk to him. Next week, I'll let you know what happens.

The session ends nicely, and both go on their merry way with smiles. What do you think the session will be like next week? If dumb luck does not come in and rescue poor Maurice, it could end up a disaster.

You see, SAM and the EA are always on the lookout for trouble. When Maurice first met his therapist, SAM was on alert and Maurice felt anxious. Over time, SAM and the EA began to relax, and anxiety reduced or even subsided in the sessions. This change can lull both the therapist and client into the illusion of a client's readiness to tackle the problem they came to therapy to address. However, this is usually wrong.

Our first job as a therapist is to build rapport and create a safe space for clients. Once they feel safe, anxiety often does come down. The problem is, this is not enough to change a person's whole anxiety-related paradigm, especially not with the issue we most fear. The moment they leave our small cocoon of tranquility, SAM goes back on the alert. Maurice could very well skip to work feeling great, believing he will achieve his dream of more money, only to take a face-plant once in the presence of the boss. Even if he is able to talk to his boss, going on the steam of belief borrowed from the therapist, he will undoubtedly notice that his body is not at all the same level of relaxed with the boss as with the therapist.

There are other consequences to this. Maurice might conclude the therapist was inept for thinking he was ready. Or he may think himself the one incompetent. In either case, progress may be set back some or stopped altogether.

What went wrong?

The therapist skipped the first step in anxiety treatment, namely, treat the experience of anxiety itself. If this does not make sense to you, you are in good company. Most people say they treat anxiety when what they really treat are the theoretical models of what happens outside of therapy. What was being treated in Maurice's situation was the cause of the anxiety, not the anxiety itself. In this section, we will discuss the first step (which is really what the entire treatment section of the book is about—laying solid foundations and accomplishing beginning steps of treatment).

What Was That Again?

By way of review, there are two primary ways to upset SAM (or ignite the amygdala). Most of us are intimately familiar with the slower, more cognitive path. Because of this, we begin with the road less traveled and will spend time analyzing the fast path.

Remember this?

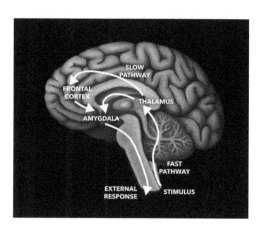

Remember our friend the thalamus? If you recall, the fast path refers to times when known threats, as tagged by the thalamus, send "Danger, Will Robinson!" signals directly to the amygdala. In such cases, the information will not have enough time to pass through our cognition before we begin to react. This can be very disconcerting, especially when the thalamus has been taught in error, or what was fearful is no longer a danger and yet the amygdala reacts as if it is a current threat. Therefore, it can be helpful to learn a few of the common triggers.

The Trigger Diary

As you saw in chapter six when Jimmy moved to Istanbul, he had many experiences most of us would call fearful. However, most of them were anxiety based and not fear based, as there was no need for flight or fight. Understanding how this works now, let's take note of the common reasons people enter treatment for anxiety. This is not an exhaustive list by any means, but hopefully, it is illustrative.

- Abandonment (To distinguish this from rejection, I will say this is the fear of being left utterly alone without recourse—something adults rarely, if ever, face.)
- Discomfort in Crowds/Public Speaking (Call it what it is, it is not a fear for the most part.)
- Financial Worries
- Rejection (This is the fear of not being cared for, loved, or wanted by others; adults do experience this.)
- Relationship Issues—Typical
- Relationship Issues—Abuse
- Work-Related Stress

I want you to take a long, hard look at the list above and let your mind wander. Think of at least four or five scenarios of each. Go ahead. I'll wait.

In all your scenarios, which anxiety triggers were actual threats to life and limb? If you said "Abuse in relationships," then you hit the nail on the head. Remember, I am not saying the other things are not life-altering, monumental, substantial, and often incredibly painful experiences. I am simply saying, we do not need to allow or put our biology in charge of the response to those issues, and we do not need to react to them in fight or flight. Instead, we need to use our minds and spirits to help us choose problem solving, people skills, and distress tolerance.

The thing is, we don't know this. I mean, it is not readily taught in this manner. Therefore, most of us are on autopilot and live subject to our neurological and biological whims. This is no slam on anyone. I was a therapist for years before I realized I was doing the same thing, and to this day, if I am not mindful, I will still succumb. I teach this almost every day and even read all the time about the dangers of living according to the brain and emotions, yet I still struggle.

Thankfully, you do not need to know the source of the trigger (in other words, *why* you are so discombobulated by public speaking or asking someone on a date). You simply need to become aware in the present moment that you are reacting to something from the past that is not a true threat—at least not anymore.

For example, every time Cynthia asked her parents for money to buy something she needed, they read her the riot act about how inconvenient and expensive she was to them. In the present day, when she wants to ask her boss for some time off (something she needs), she feels mortified and almost paralyzed at the very thought of having to ask. She may not have any idea why it is so hard. No matter . . . Cynthia needs simply to notice the emotion and the dread and ask herself the reason for it in the present moment.

For now, the important thing to understand is that the brain will adhere like white on rice to the rules established in the files if it thinks them necessary for safety and efficiency. Living at the mercy of our baser, biological instincts has a high cost. Over time, we feel used, abused, and mistreated by life in general. When this happens, most people self-medicate. Read the last sentence again. Did you see it? Most people. If you (or those you work with) fall in the category of self-medicator, you (or they) are not alone, stupid, crazy, or bad . . . you (or they) are simply trying to solve a pain problem. Join the club!

Tryin' to Heal Thyself

Okay, so now you know (if you haven't all along) that most (if not all) of your maladaptive coping techniques were developed to keep you safe and efficient. Sad, lonely, anxious, unhappy people are not very safe or efficient. If you woke up with a terrible headache but wanted to go to work, you would understandably and wisely search for something to reduce the pain, maybe some headache medicine, some breakfast, or a quick jog on the treadmill. You know to do this from common sense or experience.

What about emotional and psychological pain? It is still pain. It is still a problem to solve, and the brain—left to its own devices—will begin the hunt for a solution. Knowing what some of these solutions are can be helpful and insightful. Here, again, is by no means an exhaustive list of self-medicating techniques:

- Avoidance
- Distraction (binge-watching Netflix, gaming addiction, etc.)
- Overeating or eating disorders
- Relationship addiction
- Self-harm and parasuicidal gestures

- Substance use and abuse
- Unhelpful self-soothing behaviors (risky sex, gambling, shopping, etc.)

As with the other list above, I would like you to take a minute and think of various examples of each of these. What do they all have in common?

When everything is boiled down to basics, every one of these behaviors has the intention of either reducing or inciting emotional responses. And they work, at least for the short term.

In the long run, however, things begin to fall apart. After years of ineffectual responses to pain we do not even recognize as legitimate, our biology tends to choose one of two courses. Our emotions either shut down or explode in a chaotic cacophony of sensations—or both at different times. Both are meant to jar us into paying attention so that the underlying problem can be addressed. However, in our pursuit-of-happiness mentality, we have learned to shun all things not leading to bliss and therefore misunderstand the signals.

Take another look at the list now. Can you see which behaviors might fall into which course? For example: is shopping a calm-or-stuff-the-too-big-emotion tactic or a let's-get-this-neurotransmitter-party-started technique? What about substance use? Risky sex? Avoidance? As you work to treat others (or yourself) for anxiety and the host of other situations tempting you to indulge in self-medication, knowing which techniques you lean into might help you see whether absence or abundance of emotion is the culprit.

You may now want to ask, "Okay, so if I have too much emotion, what do I do?" or "If I'm numb and dead inside, what's the prescription then?" An in-depth conversation about this is beyond the scope of this book. Suffice it to say, for either case you need to learn emotion regulation, which falls under the category of problem-solving skills. Anxiety, depression, trauma, and other disorders tend to include a problem with the intensity, duration, frequency, and direction of our emotions. Mitigating these issues is the goal of cognitive and experiential treatment.

For our purposes today, the problem-solving, emotion-regulation skill we will learn is exposure therapy. First, however, we have some awareness raising and monitor creating to do.

How Bad Do You Really Feel?

I lead an anxiety group for several years. I often opened these sessions with a short, round-robin check-in where I said, "Tell me where your anxiety is today." I gave no measuring stick for this. I wanted people to express themselves in whatever manner they chose. Over the years, I received a plethora of interesting responses, everything from "I'm all over everywhere" to "I'm kind of orange and green today." By far, however, the most common response was a number on an arbitrary one-to-ten intensity scale, where one was calm and ten was all-out panic.

While this scale may initially seem helpful, it did very little for me as an observer and care provider. I could not count the number of times I saw a completely still, apparently placid person whisper something about being at a ten, while another excessively fidgety, sweaty, eyes-roaming-back-and-forth person declared they were not anxious at all—a "big ol' zero." Needless to say, I scratched my head a few times.

I am glad such intensity scales exist because they are an attempt to put the unspeakable into words. However, I see two major problems here. First of all, the goal is not to be afraid of anxiety. If the focus is on how intense the emotion is, then the goal often becomes reducing the sensation, and believe it or not, to focus there is counterproductive. Also, most people with mental illness will attest that other people don't "get it." I am not surprised. For the most part, the experience of anxiety, depression, and even trauma is invisible. Therefore, we need not only a way for a person to know what is happening within them, but for those around them to understand as well. Enter the SUDS chart.

SUDS stands for ***Subjective Units of Distress Scale***. The random scale listed above is not a SUDS scale, in my humble opinion. It is an intensity scale, and it varies from person to person and situation to situation. Although still utilizing the one-to-ten principle, the SUDS chart presented here is standardized, and therefore relatable.

There are many ways to establish a SUDS chart—please feel free to use your creativity, provided you do not lose the goal of making the chart usable to both the client and yourself. Looking at a serene person who calls themselves a ten is simply not helpful to anyone. For them, it instills a fear of emotion, as it implies an inability to tolerate the least amount of uncomfortable internal stimulus. For the onlooker, it is meaningless when it comes to understanding or predicting.

To help you start, let's create a standardized SUDS chart. Instead of focusing on intensity of emotion, we want people to notice their ability to maintain control of their ship. Olympic athletes in competition, public speakers, and people on dates with their long-time crushes may feel intense emotion but perform well. In these cases, the emotions subside relatively quickly without enduring mental ruminations. What we are trying to target are those who cannot manage their thinking and/or behavior.

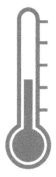

To illustrate this, take out a piece of paper and draw a thermometer (or a vertical line).

Add in five evenly spaced notches. Label each notch with even numbers from zero to ten. Zero will be at the bottom and ten at the top. Each notch represents a level of distress. It is important to note that this does not indicate level of arousal. The intensity of the emotion is not the primary focus. The goal is to notice the distress, which for our discussion indicates the level of difficulty in managing the brain and body.

Once you have created a SUDS chart, label it with typical experiences, thought types, and body sensations experienced at each level. Here is an example:

0 = No Distress: This would be a state of complete calm both in mind and body. One could be asleep, perhaps on a blanket at the beach, or blissfully watching a fire while roasting marshmallows at camp.

2 = Alert, Feeling Pleasant: Here, the person is up and active. Maybe they are baking cookies with their children, working successfully at an occupation they love, or having a conversation with a friend over tea.

4 = Mild Distress, Manageable: This is when the person knows something is off, but they are in control of their thinking and behavior. Perhaps this is during rush hour traffic, giving a presentation on a new product at work, or meeting someone for a blind date. (Note: Control does not mean they have no stressful thinking. It simply means they are not overtaken by it. They may or may not have any troublesome emotions or action urges.)

6 = Moderate Distress, Thinking Impaired: At this point, we start to run into trouble. Something is definitely wrong, and now they are losing the ability to manage their thinking. Ruminations and obsessions start at this point. This could be running the scene of a fight with a loved one over and over in their head, overanalyzing every single detail of a project for which they received criticism, or endlessly catastrophizing over a fight that might happen with a sibling.

8 = Significant Distress, Behavior Impaired: When a person reaches this level of distress, they can no longer manage their behavior. This is when a person is acting contrary to their typical nature—shouting something they do not want to say at a loved one, perhaps throwing things, or chasing someone down a hallway who has asked them for a break. This may also be when a person self-harms, though it could be done volitionally, as well.

10 = Panic/Dissociation: This is the highest level of distress. The person's brain checks out completely or they panic. A person could freeze at this point as well. This usually occurs during trauma or a panic attack.[3]

The beauty of the standardization is in having a way to measure what is happening with the person in a way both they and another person can understand. The subjective aspect comes from what each individual would put at each point of the chart. What may be a four for one person could be a two or a six for someone else. Therefore, after learning the points of the chart, it is a good idea to fill it out with your own subjective experience. It can be beneficial to include the following for each point along the scale:

1. A personal experience at the corresponding level ("On the beach in Maui last July.")
2. The type of thinking you remember having ("My mind was empty," or "I had slow and pleasant thoughts," or "My thoughts were racing.")
3. Any body sensations you can remember ("Soft and relaxed muscles," or "Quick pulse and rapid breathing," or "Clammy skin and nausea.")

If you are a care provider working with someone, it is of utmost importance you watch the person as they describe each level. You will generally notice one of two things. As the scale increases, they either become more animated and/or verbose in their descriptions, or they become less so. Creating a scale like this gives insight into how you or another person behaves or thinks and what physical

---

[3] For more examples and related worksheets, see https://bit.ly/3cutW0W.

tells they may have when approaching dangerous territory. This is necessary if you plan to engage in any kind of exposure therapy.

Once the general SUDS is completed, you may consider creating a separate chart for the presenting issue. A partial example is given later in this chapter.[4]

Calming & Grounding

Another crucial step to take before attempting to work on anxiety tolerance is to learn how to manage your brain and body during stress. There are many ways to do this. Two main categories are calming/relaxation and grounding.

Calming/Relaxation refers to reducing muscle tension and sensory overload in the body. This may include slowing of breathing, thinking, and speech as well as voluntary muscle contraction and release. It may even involve light aerobic exercise. It often depends on the system (sympathetic/parasympathetic) activated at the moment.

Grounding refers to bringing oneself back into the body and feeling connected to self and environment. This is something someone needs to do when they are dissociated or reacting out of trauma. Trauma reactions include any response in the present moment initiated by a memory trigger of an experienced trauma or fear of a future one.

For clarity and simplicity, I will refer to these as brain/body management techniques. There are a plethora of these available on the internet. My personal preference, however, is those involving both physical and mental processes so the brain and body engage together. This is one of the best ways to help the mind come back online.

Here are some examples of brain/body management techniques:

---

[4] For more examples and related worksheets, see https://bit.ly/3cutW0W.

54321: (Calming/Relaxing/Grounding) In this technique, you use a mindful awareness of your environment by listing: five things you can see, four things you feel (through your skin, not emotionally), three things you can hear (or would like to hear), two things you can smell (or would like to smell), and one thing you can taste (or would like to taste).

Four-Square Breathing: (Calming/Relaxation) Here, a person engages in diaphragmatic breathing in a four-part, systematic way. For example, they breathe in deeply to the count of four, hold their breath for a count of four, breathe out for a (longer and slower) count of four, and then hold again for a final count of four. This is repeated until the person feels in control again. It is best if the person can draw a box in the air to match the counting.

Safe-Place Imagery: (Calming/Relaxing/Grounding): This takes some learning and practice, but it involves creating a safe-place image in your brain, such as a beach, or a cabin in the mountains, or on one of the rings of Jupiter (need not be a real place, just one you can imagine). No one but you (and maybe God or a pet) can join you without your permission, and there you use all your senses to imagine safety and to do activities (such as fishing or decorating). For any negative thinking, you create a container to which to banish them.

Once you or someone you work with has an understandable way to convey their distress and you have seen them effectively use methods to reduce their physical distress, they may be ready for the technique of focus for this section: exposure therapy.

Exposure Therapy: Learning to Control the Ship

You are the owner and pilot of your vessel—you know, the thingamajig you walk around in all day. Sometimes, it does not feel that way. Okay . . . often it does not feel that way. Emotions overload, and thoughts swirl around at the speed of light. It can feel daunting. However, the truth remains that we have more power than we think we do. The more we can do to keep the body and brain at optimal functioning, the more we will feel the sense of control. This section is about one way to reduce anxiety and therefore improve our sense of well-being.

As this book is meant to capture what is taught in my seminars, exposure therapy will be the method I share. This will not be a full and robust treatment of the technique. My goal here is to lay a foundation for its use, help you understand the first step in anxiety treatment, and to whet your whistle for more information. If you find the ideas here intriguing, please do continue to learn and practice. But do not add "exposure therapist" to your business card just yet!

The first thing to understand is there are several types of exposure therapy.

In-Vivo Exposure: This is when treatment is applied to something occurring in the present moment. For example, a person with an OCD-based contamination fear comes out of the bathroom, and you ask them not to return to the bathroom to wash again. In this scenario, they are exposed to the dreaded experience in the moment.

Imagery/Virtual-Reality Exposure: This is when a person uses their imagination or a virtual-reality device to conjure up the dreaded issue.

Interoceptive Exposure: This is when a feared physical sensation (such as the emotion of anxiety or frustration) is conjured up so it can be addressed.

The type of exposure on which I will elaborate in this section will be interoceptive.

In addition to the various kinds of exposure, there are three major *paces*:

Systematic Desensitization: This generally moves the slowest and is often used with phobias. Exposure begins at the lowest possible level and is done in a slow, stepwise manner, calming the person between each iteration and repeating steps until they no longer register any anxiety.

Graded Exposure: This is when a perceived fear is ranked, and the therapist starts work at mid-level. The person is still calmed at each interval along the way.

Flooding: This is when the therapy starts at the highest level of fear and stays with it until the anxiety reduces. I do not advise anyone to attempt this for any reason without significant training.

The pace on which I will instruct is graded exposure (hence the use of the SUDS chart). To sum up, we will learn about graded, interoceptive exposure.

Our Friend Maurice

People usually present for anxiety treatment in one of two ways. The first are those who appear anxious with you in the office, at least when talking about their particular issue. The second are those who appear cool as a cucumber when with you. The first type of person is relatively easy, but the second . . . that's another story. More to come.

The method itself has these three key steps:

Step One: Determine the halfway point for the issue and begin there.

Step Two: Stay with that level of situation until they have regained control.

Step Three: Repeat the exercises until they can maintain thinking and behavioral control.

To demonstrate the technique, what follows are two possible scenarios using our friend Maurice, who wanted to ask his boss for a raise. In the first example, Maurice is easily anxious from simply talking about the issue. In the second, the therapist will need to irk Maurice a bit. In both cases, rapport has been built, the therapist knows Maurice is safe, brain-body education has taken place, and he has learned the general SUDS chart and grounding skills. They also created a problem SUDS chart—meaning they ranked the issue that brought him into therapy. Here is a section of Maurice's problem chart:

8=Asking for a raise (Could not manage to speak and would shake uncontrollably)

6=Asking for a vacation (would ruminate and worry afterward)

4=Talking to the boss in the break room (can manage his thoughts and behaviors but it is unpleasant)

2 . . .

Nervous Maurice

Therapist: So nice to see you today, Maurice! As you know, we will start our exposure practice today.

Maurice: (sheepishly) Yeah. I thought so.

Therapist: I think you were going to tell me what it was like for you to talk to your boss and why you feel it gives you so much trouble. Before we start, though, can you tell me where you are on the SUDS chart?

Maurice: (looking at the chart) Oh, I don't know. Probably a 3.5. (wringing hands as he speaks)

Therapist: (makes a note of his response) All right. Go on.

Maurice: (clearing his throat, pulling at his collar, and speaking with a shaky voice) My boss is a bit of a meanie. He hardly says three words to us most days. (clears throat again and then pauses, as if trying to figure out where to go) Uh . . . I don't know. I just know that he is mean and does not say much. I feel nervous around him. He is mean, and—

Therapist: (notices the repetition of words indicating difficulty forming thoughts, makes a quick note of the topic, and then raises a hand to get Maurice's attention) Maurice. I'm sorry to interrupt. You seem to be struggling to gather cour thoughts, which means you are up around a six. Let's stop for a minute and do your grounding technique, the 54321. Remember that? Can you tell me five things you see in the room?

(Maurice complies with the request)

Therapist: (asks for four things Maurice can feel through his skin, three things he can hear, and then stops) How are you doing now?

Maurice: (wide-eyed) Wow. That was helpful. I'm certainly in control. I'd say a solid three. I don't feel as shaken up now. What I wanted to say is that my boss intimidates me, and I fumble words when I try to talk to him.

Therapist: Excellent work! Yes. You see how stopping and grounding yourself brings down the intensity of the emotion so you can think? The idea is that you will catch yourself in the future. Now, keep going with what you wanted to say.

(Maurice is impressed because his brain cleared, and his body felt better.)

Points to note:

1. The therapist identified the SUDS score before, during, and after the exposure.

2. The target was the loss of control caused by the emotion of anxiety—not the content of what he was saying.
3. The therapist interrupted and suggested a grounding technique.

The therapist will continue to interrupt Maurice until he starts catching himself amping up and does his own grounding until the content no longer causes him to lose control.

Content Maurice

Therapist: So nice to see you today, Maurice! As you know, we will start our exposure practice today. I know you struggle with anxiety at work, but you seem to be fine when you are here with me. Where are you on the SUDS chart?

Maurice: A big, fat zero!

Therapist: Wonderful! Remember that you need to maintain control of your thoughts and behaviors. My job is to help you learn how to do that. There are many ways to accomplish this, but this way seems pretty good to start. In the box next to your chair is a box with little strips of paper in it. Please take one and answer the question as if you are giving a speech.

Maurice: (acts amused) All righty! (takes paper from box) Why should I be president? Well, that is easy! I know a whole lot more about how to run the cou—

Therapist: (looking down at her notepad but eying Maurice in her periphery, she interrupts) Stand up.

Maurice: (confused, but still amused, smirks) Uh . . . okay. (stands up) I'm not sure where I was. Oh . . . I know a lot more about how to run the country than most people I've seen try. In fact, I—

Therapist: (continuing to look at her notepad) Stand on one foot.

Maurice: (confused and starting to look and feel a bit flustered) What? Okay. (stands on one foot and continues) I used to be president of my chess club in high sch—

(Therapist stands up and walks to her desk. Rattles papers and drawers while Maurice is talking. Maurice stops, and therapist instructs him to keep going.)

Maurice: (frustrated and confused, grimacing) What is this? Umm . . . I don't understand.

Therapist: (appearing uninterested) Keep going.

Maurice: I don't understand. I was president in high school . . . umm . . . (starting to wobble on one foot)

Therapist: Jump up and down.

Maurice: Huh? I don't understand.

Therapist: (returns to her seat) Okay, sit down. Where are you on the SUDS now?

Maurice: (a spark of understanding comes over his face) Oh . . . well, I was really starting to chew you out in my head, so I guess up close to a six!

Therapist: Great work! Take a deep breath. Remember that safe place we created? Go there and tell me a couple of things you hear.

(Maurice takes a deep breath and closes his eyes. After a few seconds, he shares some things he hears in his imaginary safe place.)

Therapist: What would you take in there to taste?

Maurice: I love pizza. I would have pizza.

Therapist: Where are you now?

Maurice: (takes a deep breath) I am back down, probably a two. Now that I know what you're doing, it was kind of fun.

Therapist: You did not seem to think so a few minutes ago. What did you notice in your body through this exercise?

Maurice: I felt my dander go up, and then the exercise of the safe place brought it back down.

You see how this works? You have to find ways to conjure up the uncomfortable feeling—and if you remember the regulation systems in the body, a person in up-regulation is dominant for fear and rage. This means, essentially, you do not have to make your client anxious—irritation will work as well to create a situation where your client can learn the ability to reduce an uncomfortable emotion.

The whole idea here is for them to mindfully notice an uncomfortable emotion in the office with you. They must have a way to regain control of mind and body and eventually learn to do this unprompted. Any grounding technique will be fine. Give them time to practice and learn it.

In the instance of content Maurice, the therapist would have to be skillful, wise, and creative in how they do this. Perhaps ask them to refrain from smoking for a few hours before the session. Maybe send them on their weekly grocery shopping trip but have them visit two or three stores and stand in the longest lines, all an hour or two before coming to the session. I find the speech prompt the easiest, but if you have to repeat it, you have to up the ante by doing more unexpected things. Remember, the brain is an anticipation engine. If they have a good rapport with you and you do something unexpected, it is likely to get a rise out of them. Choosing what to do is an art though.

You can see that the therapist must be mindful and alert. You will spend weeks before you attempt an exposure exercise. If you do the SUDS right, they will ease up the ranks and not explode. Use wisdom. Spend a few months familiarizing yourself with the SUDS before you attempt exposure. Then, go slowly. Maybe practice on friends and family members. Teach them the SUDS and then simply interrupt them now and then and make a guess as to where they are on the scale.

Again, you are not an exposure therapist because of this book or the training. Keep learning. The goal is to treat the experience of anxiety before anything else. Once you are sure that what you have taught has been learned—meaning you see them reduce their distress right in front of you—only then send them out for homework.

With Maurice's example, perhaps go back to the original problem SUDS chart and ask Maurice to talk to his boss in the break room for three or four minutes and then report back. That is, if you are sure he can manage himself that long. The surest way for a person to stay anxious is to avoid what provokes anxiety. Do not give homework that allows this to happen. Also be on the lookout for those who think they are cured after one (or so) session! The client should stay with the activity long enough to show that the lowered anxiety/higher level of control is the new normal.

To sum up this section, remember—when we say we treat anxiety, it needs to be the actual experience of anxiety. We do ourselves no favors when we do not see our clients practice. Whatever your method, the idea is to help clients notice the experience of anxiety and mindfully address it in the current moment. A threat analysis, talking to the family-in-the-brain member, guided safe-place imagery, and a variety of other activities may accomplish this as well.

We have only scratched the surface here. Whichever way you decide to address anxiety in your practice, exposure therapy is in play when a person stays in the experience of the dreaded feeling until control is regained and they are no longer disturbed. It takes time and effort, but it pays off!

Tips & Tricks (For the Journey of Recovery)

It may sound kind of funny, but many people waste a lot of valuable time working on problems that are not *the* problem. We have talked about the first step in anxiety treatment as treating anxiety itself. This is so obvious as to be completely overlooked. Now, think about couples who fight over not putting a dish away or coming home late for dinner without calling. By themselves, these can be frustrating, but the true issue usually comes from the underlying problem. For example, when your partner does not put the dishes away, it is not the dirty dish, but the extra work it causes you that makes you feel uncared for. If you think about it, the true problems with others usually come from feeling uncared for, unheard, forgotten, and/or insulted. Complete this list with your own and think of a few difficult interactions you have had. What was the real problem?

Chapter Challenge Questions (Cortex Focus)

1. Create a list of your personal triggers as best you know them. Do you know where any of them originated? Are any still applicable in the present moment? Think carefully. Do you really need that reaction? Why or why not? Journal about this.

2. Create your own SUDS chart. Share it with someone safe and trusted. Journal about the experience.

Go Deeper (Somatic Focus)

Mindfulness/Awareness Activity. Set a timer on your phone or pick set times throughout the day to check in with yourself. Where are you on the SUDS chart? Check in with all your senses. Are you in control of your thoughts and behaviors? If something is going awry, what do you think would help? Try out solutions you imagine.

CHAPTER NINE

The Slow Path: Dealing with Cortex-Based Anxiety

What's Wrong with Cognitive Behavioral Therapy?

THE SHORT ANSWER to the question above is: nothing. By having a larger focus on the somatic treatments, I do not mean to imply anything negative about cognitive behavioral therapy (CBT). CBT is a wonderful treatment modality. I use it nearly every session. Nothing is wrong with it. It is simply not enough.

Years of clinical research have demonstrated that CBT is a robust, tried-and-true method of helping people with a variety of mental illnesses and distressing life situations. If anything goes wrong in the actual execution of CBT, it is typically due to the training (or lack thereof) of the therapist. Some may learn about cognitive distortions or the skill of reality testing and from then on package themselves as CBT therapists. Not so, *mon cherie*.

Therefore, it is not CBT itself that presents an issue, but the fact that we have this huge apparatus attached to our heads—our bodies! (Grin). We have two sides to our brains and two processing systems. This means that we must *always* employ techniques to treat the discomfort in the body as well as the igniting and erroneous thoughts of the brain. Despite what may have been thought before, you cannot simply think your way out of anxiety.

To be successful at executing CBT methods, it is important to develop the ability to see multiple entry points into someone's way of thinking and then ask strategic questions to unlock understanding. Truly great CBT therapists are tactically inquisitive, not directive.

In that vein, rather than teach you anything at all about CBT, a topic with which therapists are often inundated, I want to provoke you to focus on strategy, and I wish to convey the following two principles:

1. The entire goal at the beginning of cognitive treatment needs simply to be moving people off a particular neural pathway in the brain.
2. We must accomplish this with the utmost dignity, respect, and finesse—we cannot lead others where we ourselves have not gone. We can simply help them see the destination exists and help them find their way.

This is far, far easier said than done. Once flawed thinking in yourself and others becomes apparent, it is easy to become prescriptive. We say things such as "Think about something else" or "You/I shouldn't think like that." Thankfully, it is not our job to tell people what to think. Let's see what happens when we try that approach.

If You Say So . . . I Guess

Ahh, affirmations. A favorite tool for therapists everywhere! And yet . . .

What you are about to read is about as real as it gets. People everywhere are stuck in faulty thinking because society struggles so much with saying what is real and true, *nonjudgmentally*. Remember, the brain is for safety and efficiency. Without mindful attention, our brains will tag every outlier as the enemy. This results in erroneous thinking. We are *all* subject to this. Everyone. No one escapes.

A long time ago, a man named Paul of Tarsus, who spent much of his life studying and meticulously and vehemently living a particular religious philosophy, was radically changed by an encounter with Jesus. Paul wrote something I have always found comforting. The New Testament may not be everyone's cup of tea, but think of it in this manner—this man wrote this over two thousand years ago.

"We demolish arguments and every pretension that sets itself up against the knowledge of God, and *we take captive every thought* to make it obedient to Christ." (The apostle Paul to the church at Corinth, 2 Corinthians 10:5.)

As you can see by my added emphasis, I want you to notice that Paul said our thoughts are to be taken captive. Paul was a highly educated man having sat under some of the greatest minds of his time. He had been in touch with Jesus and the early church world, and yet he did not say we were not to have negative, self-defeating, erroneous, or off-color thoughts. Stop whatever you are doing (after you finish reading this sentence), sit, and ponder that a few minutes. Does that not change everything in relation to your thought world? So many people spend years beating on themselves for even having a negative thought. Paul indicates here that God Himself had the notion that judgmental and unhelpful thoughts *will* happen and are, in fact, *not* the problem. The problem arises from buying into the thoughts and allowing them to push us toward unhelpful thoughts and actions.

Whatever your spiritual bent, the principle applies: the job is not to flog yourself for erroneous thinking, but simply to notice and capture the thoughts and work to bring them in line with your values and who you truly want to be.

Wow! Seems CBT predates even Beck and Ellis. Way to go, Paul!

This in mind, it makes sense to want to change inaccurate thinking without the self-abasement we often experience in the process. When we move toward helping others, though, it is beneficial to keep an eye on pride and arrogance in order to avoid the pitfall of believing we can change another person's mind simply by the use of a technique, a formula, or telling what to think. Surely we can learn things from each other. Being third-party observers is the greatest asset a therapist, mentor, or helper has. There *are* times to be directive, but in matters of method and technique rather than heart issues. What I mean is—thinking comes, at least in part, from our core beliefs. Without full understanding and consent, we cannot take charge of or direct someone else. They will resist.

I digress.

Let's return to affirmations. I hope you have decided to let yourself off the hook for having negative or unhelpful thinking. Even so, we do not want those types of thoughts to remain. Typically, an affirmation is usually the positive opposite of a negative statement. For example, if a person says, "I am stupid," the affirmation would be "I am smart." Or, if they say, "I am worthless," the affirmative response would be "I have worth." This is simple enough, right?

What, though, is the affirmation for "I am ugly"?

Worse yet, what if you have a seventy-five-pound person sitting in your office saying, "I am fat"? What do you have them say to themselves then? Thinking of myself, I wonder who am I to impose my beliefs and value system on someone else? I cannot simply tell these people to walk around saying "I am pretty" or "I am skinny" to themselves.

We know this. Therefore, affirmations can sometimes take

a more constructive form of the negative statement. Something more like "I can make healthy choices" or "I have inner beauty." This is a start, but can you see that the problem lies in trying to convince another person to believe the way we do? I have my own subjective understanding of the world based on fifty years of experience, perceptions, and thoughts. CBT, at its core, knows that I cannot simply implant a thought into another person. It must be done by building the associated schema around it. Affirmations, if constructed incorrectly, may never accomplish this.

Therefore, we must understand the best job for an affirmation is to move a person off a neural pathway. It may be a seed that will eventually sprout a foundation for new beliefs—but that will come only after a faithful connection to the affirmation giver and/or a tremendous amount of repetition and exploration. It is best not to start with that end in mind.

Practically speaking, then, listen to yourself and others, and if you hear negative self-talk, use affirmations simply as a way to try out another pathway.

Take a Different Road

Janice had had enough. She finally bit the bullet and called a therapist. When it was just her sister on her case for her weight, that was fine. However, she was convinced she lost her chance at her dream job because of it, and she was just done. She needed help, and she knew it.

In the first session, the nice lady, Linda, with the kind and searching eyes, blond bob, and endless smile, sat in the satiny chair in front of her, legs crossed, pen and notepad in hand. Janice was at a loss. She knew if she said what she really thought, this sweet girl would think she was crazy and lock her away.

To avoid all of that, she proceeded to tell Linda that her troubles revolved around work-related anxiety. She felt she could not

present her best self in an interview. Two or three sessions passed.
Linda probed for history, and Janice stuck to her cover story.

We are funny, aren't we? We don't have the whole story here,
but you may have been able to tell early on that more was up with
Janice than she was admitting. How is it, then, she expects Linda to
help her? This goes on all the time. Janice does not want to say out
loud to another human the actual words that will bring healing.
Linda, thankfully, knows this.

Something surprising happened during the fourth session.

> **Janice:** (actually feeling desperately alone and unseen)
> It has been nice talking to you. When I come here, I feel
> better. It makes me want to get out there and try harder.
> I think I'm ready to apply for another job.
> **Linda:** (pausing to think) Really? I don't think you are.
> **Janice:** (shocked and taken aback) Oh? Really? I
> thought things were going well.
> **Linda:** Janice, you have not yet told me the reason you
> are here.
> **Janice:** (squirming a bit in her chair) What do you
> mean? I told you the first day. It's all we have been work-
> ing on so far.
> **Linda:** It is all *you* have been working on. I have sim-
> ply been listening, asking questions, and observing. You
> are not here because you are nervous about interviews,
> are you? (Unexpectedly, Janice begins to cry and shake.
> Her eyes dart to the floor and stay there, fixed, almost
> unblinking. Linda sits in silence, allowing Janice to find
> her thoughts. Once she does, the words pour out.)
> **Janice:** In high school, I won prom queen. I was one
> hundred and fifteen pounds sopping wet. After college
> and a big, heart-wrenching breakup, I figured out that
> food could be a friend. I hate myself. I'm ugly and hid-
> eous. I know my last interview bombed—not because

I am not skilled at what I do and say, but because I could not even bring myself to bother to comb my hair. I mean, what for? They are going to take one look at me, consider me a joke, and move on. I am not anxious in interviews. I'm just fat and ugly.

What do you think would be the right course of action for Linda at this stage? If she is like many therapists out there, she will work to comfort Janice and help her see her strengths. What if Linda were to prescribe an affirmation?

> **Linda:** Oh, I'm sure it's not that. There are lots of great features about you! I doubt anyone would avoid hiring you simply because of your outer appearance. Last week, you told me you liked the color of your hair. It is a beautiful auburn. I bet if you spend some time focusing on how beautiful your hair is, you will start to notice other areas of beauty. You just need to raise your confidence so you can go in there with your head held high. I bet it had more to do with your confidence than your appearance!

BEEP . . . Thank you for playing. No.

Do you see some problems with Linda's approach? Although she caught on to Janice's all-or-nothing or overgeneralizing cognitive errors, she was prescriptive, dismissive, and plain wrong. You bet your butter some people would reject a perfectly skilled candidate based solely on their looks. Janice is no dummy. She knows how the world works. That is not the problem. Janice finding her "one in eighteen billion-ness" and bringing that into play is the goal.

What if Linda took a different road—the road of truth telling? What might that look like? Fasten your seat belts . . .

Linda: (allowing herself to feel a bit of Janice's pain) Thank you.

Janice: (confused) For what?

Linda: For telling me the true story. If I understood right, you have gained weight over the years and have given up a bit on caring for yourself. You feel that is the reason others do not want to connect with you. That is painful. Do you know why it was so difficult to tell me?

Janice: (with self-deprecating venom, staring at the floor) Because if you knew that I often order and eat an entire pizza myself at night or that my sister is right—that I'm just a worthless, fat cow—then maybe you would think I was too far gone to help. All I wanted was to feel a bit better. Talking to you—to anyone who will listen—feels better. I figured I got all I was going to get before you rejected me too.

Linda: (pausing to let Janice's words rest) Would you do me a favor? Would you look at me for a minute?

Janice: (reluctant, slowly raises her head to quickly peek at Linda) Okay.

Linda: What do you see?

Janice: I'm confused.

Linda: Look at my face. Do I look appalled?

Janice: (looking up again) Well . . . no.

Linda: My job is not to judge you. I have no doubt you arrived at where you are for legitimate reasons. You are overweight. Our society frowns on that. You are not blind, you know that. Kudos to you for being real. Now . . . what do you actually want?

Janice: (no hesitation at all) To be pretty.

Linda: (not attempting to talk her out of it) What do you think reaching that goal will entail?

Janice and Linda finish the session by brainstorming steps needed to reach Janice's goal. Along the way, Linda has to stop

Janice periodically for reality checks, and Janice responds positively because Linda has proven she listens and will not refute or attempt to simply replace Janice's thinking without exploration. Linda knows that attempting to cajole Janice into repeating positive comments to herself in the face of overwhelmingly contrary nonverbal messages will not work. Truth works. Linda's job is to help Janice find and embrace, change when possible, and accept the truth of her life.

Truth-Focus Statements

Using the example of Janice and Linda, let's learn how to create a truth-focus statement. The focus part will be explained shortly. For now, the emphasis will be on the truth aspect.

After a few more sessions and ironing out the real problem, Linda begins to help Janice find truth.

> **Janice:** (clearly agitated) I'm such a failure. A total, fat, loser failure.

Linda knows that this kind of language is not about accuracy but *impact*. Janice feels so bad in her own skin and about the slow progress of change that she is using overarching statements to describe herself. The neurons firing together on this path will lead only to a downward spiral. Janice needs to jump onto another path—and soon.

> **Linda:** You are using some pretty harsh language on yourself there. What is the real problem?
> **Janice:** (thoughtfully) I am angry for giving in to my temptations this week.
> **Linda:** Yes. That is much more accurate.

Linda spends some time educating Janice regarding the rules

and precedents she establishes in her brain when she uses the same words repeatedly. Using CBT as a base, Linda might ask Janice to look up the words she is using on herself in the dictionary. Janice is clearly not a failure or a loser, certainly not a total one of either.

Interestingly, Janice's actual problem in the moment had to do with giving in to temptation—not with her weight per se. Linda will explain to Janice that her brain listens to her, and if she tells it she is a failure and a loser, the brain has nowhere to go with that and will often simply give up trying. However, knowing that the true issue is difficulty with temptations gives a clear road forward: figure out a way to fortify healthy choices in moments of temptation.

When faced with an erroneous amygdala-activating thought, rather than prescribing a cut-and-dried or possibly condescending affirmation, try asking this question:

What is still true, but more helpful to say to yourself than that?

Think about how that might be different. Here are some possibilities.

Here's the big problem: a positive affirmation is a judgment! Yes, you read that right. According to Marsha Linehan in her DBT training videos, a judgment is a "shortcut for consequences." A person calls themselves stupid as a result of a situation, but over time, they lose sight of this if something isn't done to stop that.

Look back at the chart above. We know the negative statement will not take the client anywhere. However, can you see how the truth statement, not the affirmation, reveals the actual problem? Not studying, not having strong social skills, not liking aspects of your appearance, or realizing a person sees themselves differently than others are all issues that can be addressed. "I am smart/worthy/pretty/skinny" ends the story, and nothing much changes. What we need is to focus on and tell the truth.

Negative Self-talk	Positive Affirmation	Truth Statement
I am stupid	I am smart/ intelligent	I sometimes do not take the time I need to study
I am worthless	I have worth/value	I am socially awkward
I am ugly	I am pretty/ beautiful	I do not like how I look, especially (particular feature[s])
I am fat	I am thin/I can make healthy choices	I do not see myself the way you do

What If the Truth Hurts?

I know what you are thinking.

Whoa doggy, you sure dove deep there. In the words of the illustrious Jack Nicolson, sometimes "[People] can't handle the truth!" I mean, what on earth do I do if someone's truth is so very different from mine, or worse, hurtful (the person really is socially awkward) or dangerous (their behavior really is as bad as they say)?

Thank you for going here with me as I dig deep. I know looking at truth can be painful at times. I also hear you if you are worried about this. I mean, what if you had a seventy-two-pound grown-up person telling you they were fat? Sometimes, no matter how crafty you are at asking questions, irrationality wins, and you cannot change their mind no matter what you say or do.

I have some good news. You do not have to!

Remember, our primary goal in CBT is simply to knock a person off the path on which they have been relentlessly trodding. Step one is not to replace a person's entire belief system! All we want them to do at first, as they are slowly building trust and skills, is to consider another line of thought. Anyone who engages in negative self-talk all day long will undoubtedly feel better if they get off that path, even temporarily. If we can help people feel better in their emotional states, they are likely to be much more open to changing their thinking patterns.

Another key aspect of a vigorous course of CBT would be to use whole-brain techniques. In therapy, we spend a lot of time talking. Talking is left brain. Talking is also theory. If you want to take steps closer to experience and practice in your healing journey, then engage the visual/somatic right side. Here is an example of how I do that.

Mind as a Garden

Imagine your brain is a garden. I mean it. Go with me.

Look around. Flowers. Trees. Birdies. It's beautiful and lush.

Your attention is a water pot, and with your water pot in hand, you walk around your lovely garden watering the plants and flowers. Can you see it?

Uh oh. There are weeds in your garden.

Everything in your garden is a thought. Flowers, trees, and birdies are helpful thoughts. Weeds are unhelpful. All gardens have weeds. Yes, all of them.

What do you do with weeds? Silly question, right? You pull them up, of course! Go back to your garden. Do you see some weeds? Once you notice them, I suppose you could sit and stare at them, lamenting, "Weeds, weeds . . . there are weeds in my garden!" Sounds a bit silly though, doesn't it? Likewise, would you waste water on them? I think not.

Are we in agreement then? Don't stare at them. Don't endlessly lament them. Certainly, don't water them. Pull the lousy things out! Once you attempt this, though, you will find there are two types of weeds: easy and hard. Easy weeds come out by the roots simply by pulling them. Easy peasy. Other weeds you have to spray and dig at and pull and pull, and even when you do finally get them out, they grow back, the little buggers! Sheesh!

To have a lush, thriving garden, though—that is the work that must be done. A savvy gardener accepts the fact that weeds will grow no matter what they do. Some weeds will return. Even so, the mission is a weed-free garden. In that quest, no gardener ignores the hard weeds, and neither do they spend their days staring at the weeds in anguish. The job is never ending, and that is no reflection on the gardener. They know it simply is the way it is, and there is great satisfaction and a sense of accomplishment at learning the tricks of the trade that take them ever closer to the ultimate goal.

The Magic Questions

The above method is a great way to strategically prepare a person to do work on their thought life. Notice some key elements.

1. Everything in the garden is a thought.
2. Some thoughts are unhelpful.
3. Some unhelpful thoughts are more difficult to weed out (pun intended) than others.
4. Weeds of some sort will always grow—this is not a character flaw!

Introducing these ideas in passing can help you later when clients attempt to argue their positions. This is the art of CBT—strategically finding ways to help people see their thoughts without fear or judgment.

After creating the visual image in the brain, there is a three-step procedure that can help you begin to unravel unhelpful thoughts.

Step One: Identify the Weeds

To an untrained eye, weeds can be attractive and pass for flowers. If close attention is not paid, they will be overlooked. In all my years of practice, I've tried out a number of methods to locate negative thinking, but I have found the word "unhelpful" to be the best inroad. If I try to convince someone that a thought is wrong, bad, or even unhealthy, I receive far more pushback than I do with unhelpful. Most people can agree—even if they like their thought—that if others are pestering them about it, it is an unhelpful thought.

Therefore, the first thing to do is ask, "Please tell me some of your unhelpful thoughts." I usually take it a step further because I don't want them to tell me every random thought they have. I clarify: "Tell me unhelpful thoughts you have that start with 'I am' or 'I feel.'" I also advocate writing these down on a whiteboard so you can both be sure of what was said and not forget any.

After these statements are captured (five or six is enough), take the time you need to go back through each one to understand their history. Remember the chart from a few sections back? Here are the negative self-talk statements:

Negative Self-talk
I am stupid
I am worthless
I am ugly
I am fat

Ask the person why they feel stupid, worthless, ugly, and fat. It is incredibly important to listen and not try to change anything at this point. Validate when you can. "I can see why you think that given . . ." People with cognitive distortions are not crazy or stupid. The thoughts come from somewhere. Listening without trying to change anything allows those reasons to emerge without the person feeling less than.

Also, simply noticing what is said will help greatly with step two.

Step Two: Easy Weed or Hard Weed?

You have your list of weeds. You know where the weeds came from. Now, it is time to determine which are hard and which are easy. To do this, return to each statement and ask the following questions:

1. Is the statement true?
2. Does it help to focus on it?

Let's take each in turn.

It will not be enough most of the time to simply ask, "Is the statement true?" You will want to ask it in such a way that the answer is obviously no. For example, "I am stupid." If you ask a person, "Is that true?" they, still swimming in cognitive distortions, will often say yes. However, if you ask, "Is it really true that you are not able to learn?" then their answer is more likely to be no.

This is where your listening to the rationale of each statement is so important. You want to understand their take. If you are told that Krissy does well with writing assignments but constantly fails her tests, you will empathize and understand why she feels stupid—but is she? What is the actual problem? Most likely, she struggles to remember details for tests, or her anxiety takes over. These are solvable problems. According to *Merriam-Webster*, though, *stupid* means "unable to learn," and if that is the case, then Krissy needs to quit school and probably sit at home and stare at the wall.

I know I sound crotchety here. What I am saying is Krissy's emotional state is reflecting the need to sit at home and stare at the wall because she is telling herself she is stupid. However, she is not, so another part of her (let's call that part her right brain) says, "Hey! Wait a minute! I want to get out and have a life!" This is what we call **dissonant**. Confusion ensues, and unable to appropriately articulate the problem, Krissy feels overwhelmed and inches closer to retiring to couch-potato-ville.

You know and I know that Krissy is not stupid. The problem is that Krissy does not *noetically* know. That means you need to listen so you can ask questions that help her see. This takes time and practice. I suggest you start with family and friends. It could be fun. Just saying.

You ask, "Is it really true that you are unable to learn how to pass tests?" They say, "Well, no . . . I can learn." Yay! The answer to question one is a resounding no!

This means it is an easy weed!

When the answer to question one is no, it is an easy weed. You can simply cross it out. They outright said it is both unhelpful and untrue. Moving on.

Question two: "Well, then, does it do you any good to focus on that thought?" That's an easy no most of the time. Yay!

The majority of the statements will go this way if you are strategic in asking your questions. However, there are times when no matter how careful and tactical you are in asking, the answer will be yes.

"Given that you have been involved in treatment at eating-disorder clinics and many professionals have told you that you are underweight, is it really true that you are fat?"

"Yes."

"You say you have been married for ten years and your husband is so supportive. Your children have straight As at school, and everyone compliments you on how nice they are—is it really true that you are a bad mother?"

"Yes."

This is where we struggle. We can see very clearly how irrational their yes is. We want to yank it away and shake them. Stop for a minute though. Why would a person say yes in these cases? My guess is they either really cannot see it, have collected evidence over the years that it is true (however faulty that evidence may be), or are in denial to save themselves from a truth that feels much worse. The reasons for it are legitimate. Safety matters.

Here is where your character will be built as a therapist. You must not argue, persuade, beg, convince. You simply ask the questions and move on—because the method saves you. Here is an example.

> **Therapist:** You have told me you have worked for the same company for twelve years and have moved up the ranks regularly. However, you think you are a terrible employee. You gave this as an example of an unhelpful thought. My question is, is that statement actually true? (Question 1) Are you an all-around terrible employee?
> **Clive:** (unhesitatingly) Yes.
> **Therapist:** Okay. Thank you. If that is the case, we will make a plan to get rid of that unhelpful thought/weed. Even though you believe the statement is true, will it do you any good to focus on the thought once you create a plan to deal with it? (Question 2)

You see how that works? Question one helps to understand the level of entrenchment in the belief, and question two gives the needed permission to suggest another neural pathway to try. Remember, the goal is simply to spend some time in the flowers rather than the weeds. That's all we want. We do not need to yield to the internal push to move faster. Any constructive thought is better than where they started.

A note of caution. Please use your clinical and human judgment. If a person's erroneous belief system is in charge of their behavior and they are in danger, then a slow, methodical method will not work. Containment, hospitalization, or coping skills might be needed first. Remember, if the person is not safe, the correct response is fight (get help) or flight (get out). This technique works best with stable, non-dissociating people who have adequate social support. Take time to ensure this before you try this method.

Use this method with each of the weeds you have identified. The "plan" part could take several sessions. If the person is socially awkward, the plan could be to learn communication skills. If the person feels fat but is not, the plan could include emotion regulation and turning the mind. If they feel ugly, the plan may involve going to a makeup artist or fashion consultant. Who knows? The plan takes time to develop and execute. Right now, you simply want them off the beaten (to death) path. If they open the door to other possibilities, they may be more likely to stay on a healthier path.

Step Three: Pick a Flower

You have identified the weeds, as well as which ones are hard and which are easy. For all weeds, you must find a way to agree that it is not helpful to focus on the weeds as they are. Now, the job is to find a flower to look at instead. In other words, create a truth-based focus statement that answers the question, "What do I do if that old thought enters my mind?"

Some people will struggle with question two. At first, many people think you are asking them to give up their belief or behavior. You are not. At this stage, you are simply asking them to try out some other thought patterns. They cannot help if the thought enters their mind. They may even mull it over a while. What you want is for them to be willing to think about something else more and more of the time. Stop staring at or watering the weeds.

Help them create the truth-focus statements in column three. Remember them from above?

Truth Statement
I sometimes do not take the time I need to study
I am socially awkward
I do not like how I look, especially (particular feature[s])
I do not see myself the way you do

As a reminder, truth statements may be generated by asking, "What is still true but more helpful?"

> What is still true but more helpful than "I am stupid"?
> Example: "I struggle with math."
> What is still true but more helpful than "I am unworthy"?
> Example: "I do not feel important to my family."
> What is still true but more helpful than "I feel ugly"?
> Example: "I don't like how I look."
> What is still true but more helpful than "I am fat"?
> Example: "People do not see me how I see myself."

You see? All we want is a willingness to leave the old neural path for one that moves even slightly toward (A) an actual problem to solve and/or (B) a more constructive way to think.

The Moral of the Story

You have used both sides of the brain to create an image of a lush garden in which anyone would want to spend time. You have acknowledged that everything in the garden is a thought. You have identified weeds in the garden (unhelpful thoughts). You have listed out those weeds. You have determined which will come out easily and which may take more work. You agree to create a plan to do that work, but in the meantime, you also create a statement of focus that begins the building of a new neural pathway that will undoubtedly feel better than the old one. You have instructed the person to turn their mind to the truth-focus statement whenever they notice the old thinking—unless they are involved in the actual working of their plan.

The overall key to success in changing people's thoughts is to slow down. Changing schemas is part of the goal, but you must start with step A. Build trust and help the client imagine a new path. Most people with deeply entrenched cognitive errors cannot see them. Then, once they see them, they have to admit a whole slew of difficult things and do a lot of work to remove them. No one dances for joy at this point. Give them time. You will face less resistance if the person is able to move step by step rather than attempting to make an immediate about-face.

Tips & Tricks (For the Journey of Recovery)

We have learned we must treat the body as well as the brain and mind. However, in this chapter, we focused on thinking. Think about something you disagree about with someone you love. How did you come to the conclusion you have? What are some of the experiences you had that made you adopt the belief you have? Now, argue the opposing view with yourself. For example, suppose you believe art therapy is hokey. Perhaps you feel this way because your father laughed at your art-therapy project for school or you know insurance does not readily pay for it. Now, try to argue its positives and why it should be used. If you can learn to see things from both sides, you still may not agree, but you will find that the person holding the "weird opinion" derived theirs in just as logical and practical a manner you did. Keep this in mind when trying to help others.

Chapter Challenge Questions (Cortex Focus)

1. According to you, what is the place of thinking with regard to mental health and healing?
2. Have you used affirmations before? Did they help? What was the process? How do you feel about the statements made about affirmations in this chapter? Explain.
3. Think about a negative self-talk statement you have been making lately. For example: "I will never learn to organize my house!" Write out your rationale for that belief. Ask yourself the two magic questions. Create a plan if you need. Come up with a targeted truth-focus statement and write it on an index card. Read it proactively and when you are feeling triggered by the old thought.

Go Deeper (Somatic Focus)

Mindfulness Activity. We often struggle to know our thoughts. Choose a time when you can work uninterrupted, and find a quiet place to sit by yourself. Spend some time centering and breathing until your body feels relaxed. As you do this, imagine you are a bystander in your mind. Spend five or ten minutes simply noticing what internal actions happen in your brain and mind. Do not try to change anything. Simply notice. Do you find yourself distracted? Gently turn back. What is the content you notice? How about the feelings in the body?

Narrative Activity. Think about a difficult interaction you had with someone else. Write about the interaction, paying particular attention to the thoughts you had. Look at the thoughts. Try to recreate the story with thoughts you feel may be more accurate for the time. What do you notice?

CHAPTER TEN

Putting It all Together

WHEW! WOW! YOU did it! You read through the whole book to this point (I won't tell if you skipped a few places). Now it is time to see what all of this looks like with a practical example. First, I want to introduce you to a tool that will help you raise awareness in a way that captures both cognitive and somatic information.

Are You Aware?

At the beginning of the healing journey, most people who seek help do not really understand what is happening inside them. Remember the airplane guidance system left on autopilot? Raising awareness of what is occurring in body, mind, spirit, and relationships throughout the day is an important step toward health.

It is common to encourage this by asking clients to check in with themselves. However, this may be too vague, especially for those dealing with anxiety. Vague directions may feel overwhelming. Then, once they do check in, they may have no idea what to do with what they find, which leaves them feeling out of control.

Enter the five-point check-in, a practice developed over years and tested daily with hundreds of people at The Center: A Place of HOPE—a world-class partial-hospital program near Seattle, Washington. Within the human system, there are five key points wherein we can gain information and make adjustments to positively affect the whole. These five areas are:

1. Thoughts. Often the ruler of the system, thoughts include the information we gain from the brain (rumination, worry, memory) and mind (decision-making and metacognitions).
2. Moods. These are emotional states that have lasted at least ten minutes (sadness, happiness, fear, etc.).
3. Behaviors. These are actions we have taken in response to the moods and/or thoughts (pacing, isolating, or snippiness, for example).
4. Physical Reactions. This is how the body responds to thoughts and moods (tension, upset stomach, and headache, to name a few).
5. Environment. This is the situation we are in and the people we are with at any given time (alone at home, out at a busy concert, arguing with a sibling, and so on).

The world rushes quickly past most of us each day. The five-point check-in allows us to stop and look at what is happening in each of these areas. It is most useful to look at only small chunks of time so one can remember the information a bit easier and also cut down on trying to process too much information. Therefore, several times a day, ask yourself the following questions:

> In the last three hours, how have my thoughts been?
> Potential responses: racing, happy, sad, absent.

In the last three hours, how have my moods been?
Potential responses: happy, sad, indifferent, apathetic.

In the last three hours, how has my behavior been (or what have I been doing)?
Potential responses: snippy, engaging, withdrawn, fidgety.

In the last three hours, what has my body been like (or how have I felt physically)?
Potential responses: cold, hot, sore, energetic.

In the last three hours, what has my environment been like (or what has been going on around me)?
Potential responses: engaging, overstimulating, under-stimulating, hostile.

If a specific answer cannot be found, start with pleasant or unpleasant.

Now, imagine your answers to these questions are, respectively: ruminating, anxious, snippy, tense and hot, and isolating. What does that tell us? Well, for most, the answer is simply "I'm miserable." That would be the response to a general check-in. Knowing this alone may not be helpful. Now, we need the magic question.

After answering the five-point questions above and gathering the information, teach people to ask themselves: "What might I need?" Let's look at this by answering a few more questions. Looking back at each point, think about what your answers might be to:

If I'm having ruminating thoughts, what might I need?
Examples: a focused truth statement, a distraction, a solution to a problem.

If I'm anxious, what might I need?
Examples: exercise, a solution a problem, sleep, to play.

If I'm snippy with others, what might I need?
Examples: to make an amend, a hug, time to myself.

If I'm tense and hot, what might I need?
Examples: a massage, a bath, exercise, sleep.

If I'm isolating, what might I need?
Examples: connection, time to myself, purposeful activity.

As you can see, there is not just one answer to these. It is a bit of a quest. Therefore, it is important to say "What *might* I need?"—at least at first. Some people do not know what they need. Once they understand themselves better and feel confident in what works for them in patterned situations, they can ask more directly, "What *do* I need?"

One last note on this . . . what if the answers to the questions are good things? What if you find that you are having happy thoughts, experiencing excitement, acting friendly, and feeling calm while out at a picnic at the park on a sunny day with people you love? Then, do you still ask the "What might/do I need?" question? Yes! Absolutely. The answer then is: more of this! It is just as important to track what is going well as it is to track what is not. This is a paradigm shift for some people.

By using awareness exercises proactively and consistently, people can begin to track their patterns, notice what works, and even catch themselves feeling good!

A Simple Hack

Hack—have you heard that term before? It means "a quick way to get something done." For fun, I am including a simple whole-person hack to help integrate learning quicker—another way to bring it all together.

I call this the Labyrinth Exercise (see the link to worksheets).[5] Once a truth-focus statement has been created, have the person write it on the bottom of the worksheet. Then, a few times a day, have them trace the labyrinth while saying the statement out loud.

Why? Because the more of the brain used, the quicker something is learned. Looking at the labyrinth engages the occipital lobe. Saying it out loud and moving your hand engage the parietal and temporal lobes. Doing it in a labyrinth requires frontal lobe action. If nothing else, though, it slows the person down and forces them to say something positive a few times a day. Give it a try!

A Day in the Life

Let's put everything together with a little story.

The breeze blew through the trees on that cold autumn afternoon as Ivy sat staring out her bedroom window. Unable to stop her mind from racing and her heart from pounding through her chest, she dreaded the day to come. For as long as she could remember, she had struggled with debilitating anxiety that often led to long bouts of depression and dissatisfaction with life. She knew why. Being the only child of an angry, alcoholic father and oblivious mother had started her on a rocky foundation. Her abusive ex was just icing on the cake. Ivy did not believe there was anyone she could trust.

Yet there she was, less than an hour away from her first counseling appointment. She had finally relented after lying in bed for

---

[5] For more examples and related worksheets, see https://bit.ly/3cutW0W.

a week. Her best friend had panicked when she did not answer her phone and had come over crying and begging her to get help. So she did.

She arrived at the office, which was sparsely but nicely decorated with earth tones and blues. There was a particularly nice bird picture on the wall. Ivy liked birds and often thought about how nice it would be to fly away from the world.

A door across the room opened, and a grandmotherly woman with short, bobbed, gray hair and glasses called her name. A cold wash of dread came over her as she pulled herself up from the soft chair and padded across the floor behind the kindly lady.

"My name is Dr. Margaret Moore. You can call me Margaret, or Dr. Margaret if you prefer. Please don't call me Dr. Moore—that was my father!" she said with a crooked smile. "What brings you in to see me today?"

What proceeded was an hour of background followed by two more sessions of the same. After two or three sessions of listening and asking lots of questions, Dr. Margaret began to teach Ivy about how her brain, central nervous system, and body worked in anxiety and depression. This was surprising because Ivy had expected to hear a lot of "How did that make you feel?" as she rummaged through her messed-up past. Hanging out her dirty laundry for even an educated stranger to see was not at all appealing. This was a breath of fresh air.

Ivy learned some amazing things about herself. She learned that her brain was like a file cabinet that was managed by her frontal lobe, which Dr. Margaret referred to as the executive assistant. She learned that neural pathways formed whenever she repeated a behavior, and these pathways were how the EA retrieved things from the files. Sweet Dr. M called these pathways minions. It was fun to picture the little yellow guys running back and forth at lightning speed! Dr. M explained that memories were in the file cabinet, and in order to be retrieved in the future, each memory had a tag.

Some tags were language-based and some emotion-based. Some of Ivy's memories did not even have time tags! This meant that, for her, the memory of something long ago could feel as current as if it happened today. That explained a lot.

After teaching Ivy about her brain and body, Dr. M spent time talking about something called a SUDS chart and several grounding activities. They spent time talking about all kinds of experiences she'd had—everything from lying on the beach in Maui to fleeing from her ex in the middle of the night. Ivy learned that the intensity of the emotion was not the problem—it was the loss of connection and control of her thoughts and actions that caused problems. Dr. M said she had to learn to notice her anxiety so she could proactively address it, and had her check in several times a day, looking at five different areas of life. After not too long, Ivy noticed some patterns she had not seen previously.

For a few sessions, Dr. M let Ivy talk about all the things that bothered her in her current life, but whenever Ivy seemed to be ramping up—repeating the same thing again and again or showing physical signs of distress, Dr. M would stop her (even mid-sentence) and have her do some sort of grounding activity. Grounding was this cool thing that brought Ivy back from the abyss into her body.

More than anything, Ivy wanted to have a loving relationship with a husband, children, and maybe even a Pomeranian. She had always wanted one of those. It is difficult to care for a dog when you live alone, though, so she gave up on the idea. She had given up every idea, she came to realize as she discussed her "I am" and "I feel" statements with Dr. M. She had not realized how much of what she thought each day was not true!

Ivy felt embarrassed sometimes by all the goofy things she thought and did. Dr. M had words of kindness and compassion for that too. She introduced Ivy to the family in her brain, and Ivy began to understand that sometimes she wrestled with a Bully, other times she went future-tripping with the Worrier, but most of the time her life was run by SAM and her inner child. Ivy did not like this, but she understood, and the world started to make more sense.

After several sessions of being interrupted, it clicked for Ivy that she had the ability to reduce her anxiety. She had had no idea about this before. She had thought that emotions were always right and just did whatever they urged her to do. She had always felt helpless and never realized how truly frightening it had been to live in a body that didn't seem to like her. It had been so hard to understand and explain, but what Dr. M said made so much sense. For the first time in her adult life, Ivy felt as if she was in the present moment, confident and hopeful.

Dr. M began to assign small tasks outside the office. Say hi to someone at the bus stop. Compliment someone in the store. Learn a new hobby and join a club of other people doing that hobby. Each step was frightening, and she had to debrief it and continue to practice her grounding and thinking skills.

Six months after meeting Dr. M, Ivy was asked on a date. At first it was wonderful, but by the time she was supposed to go, Ivy panicked and canceled the date. She felt humiliated and like a complete failure. She did not want to tell Dr. M what happened, but she did.

Thankfully, Dr. M was prepared. She was not upset or disappointed in Ivy at all. Ivy learned that relapse is a part of the process. Rather than minimizing it, Dr. M expressed empathy for the situation and helped Ivy figure out what caused the fear. The next time Ivy was asked out, she accepted, went, and had a wonderful time!

Ivy and Dr. M spent three years working together. After Ivy learned how to manage her own emotions, she was able to process some of the experiences she had with her family of origin and her ex-boyfriend. It was freeing to be rid of the shame, fear, and anger. Dr. M had to remind Ivy to use her skills multiple times, but instead of feeling stupid, Ivy was grateful. She realized that everyone who has a brain is subject to the same types of struggles—sometimes in different ways and varying degrees—but we all succumb to external forces if we are not mindful.

Around the ninth month of therapy, Ivy came home from one particularly moving and helpful session and called her best friend. With tears and a full heart, she asked if she could take her friend out to her favorite restaurant to thank her for pushing her to go see Dr. M. She had never thought in a million years she could find her way out of the deep pit she had felt buried under for so many years—but she had. She knew now that she was not her brain. She was unique, special, and had assets as well as deficits . . . and by golly, she was going to use them!

Okay, okay, there was a fair amount of cheesiness in that story, but do you see the point? Adding a bit more structure to therapy early on and teaching clients about their brains, bodies, and how to manage emotional states can pave the way for more successful and long-lasting relief from the pains of anxiety, depression, and trauma. Until you deal with the physical feelings in the body, it can be very difficult to sustain progress.

Parting is Such Sweet Sorrow

Are we there yet?

Actually, yes. The time has come to go our separate ways. What an adventure this has been! I am so excited we could do this together. As we wind down and wrap up all our thoughts, I sincerely want to encourage you to never give up on the road to health. It can be bumpy, chaotic, and long—so very long. That said, it is also the best work you will ever do, full of empowerment, joy, accomplishment, warmth, adventure, and love. In short, it is worth the price you will pay because *you* are worth the price you will pay.

If, along the way, you believe I may be of any service to you, please do not hesitate to contact me. My email address is Hannah@ PotentialFinders.com. Whatever you do, please reach out and find safe people who can walk this road beside you. The message I most mean to convey is that there is hope. Your road is unique, and it may take time to find the right path. Grieving and hard work are part of the process, but they lead to lush and lavish places of abundance, where what you sow returns to you "pressed down, shaken together, and running over" (taken from the New Testament writing of Luke 6:38) and results in *Lasting Change*.

God bless you! Bye for now!

Tips & Tricks (For the Journey of Recovery)

"The best way to learn is to teach"—this is so true! If you have learned while reading this book, it could be helpful to teach others—but watch out! Those who know you, watch your life, interact with you daily, and have peer relationships with you are not likely to want to receive your teaching unsolicited. Think about times others have tried to teach you without your permission. How well did that go? If you have someone you can teach some of the principles to, please do. Otherwise, write a lesson plan you would use to show someone else.

Chapter Challenge Questions (Cortex Focus)

1. What do you think of the five-point check-in? How would you remember to do it every day?
2. As people first attempt to raise self-awareness and check in, they often do not know what they need. Why is it so hard to know what we need sometimes? Journal about it.
3. Try a five-point check-in and/or the Labyrinth activity at least two times a day for a week. What do you notice? Journal about it.

Go Deeper (Somatic Focus)

Narrative Activity. Write your own version of a "day in the life," demonstrating how you would use the skills you learned in this book. If you prefer not to write, make a collage, draw it, or sing about it.

ACKNOWLEDGMENTS

WHERE DO I begin?

First and foremost, I want to thank God for saving me—and I mean that literally, and not only for the priceless gift of salvation. I mean pulling me up off the floor, dusting me off, and putting me on the road toward a healthier life.

Back on earthly terrain, I want to especially thank my husband, Richard; my dear friend and roommate, Kelly; and the world's best in-laws, Leo and Jan, for sharing me with the country (traipsing around as I do) and the computer (especially in the final days). Thank you to Virginia—I could not have done it without all your encouragement and belief in me. Irene and John, you both have inspired me as well as encouraged me.

I am thankful for Athena Dean-Holtz of Mountain View Press for her contagious excitement at the completion of this book.

Finally, it may seem funny, and I doubt any of them will ever see this, but I want to thank Dr. Daniel Seigel, Dr. Bessel van der Kolk, Alan Shore, Bonnie Badenoch, Susan Gantt, and all the other countless people who have contributed to interpersonal neurobiology and theories such as Polyvagal theory and attachment theory. We need to keep pushing the edges and seeking not only what we know in our left brains, but also the deep noetic knowing that we each share—the golden thread, as it were, that binds us as a human family. Sir Isaac Newton said that he accomplished what he did by "standing on the shoulders of others." This is especially true for me. My main job in all of this has been science interpreter—making complicated things make sense—but I can only do that because of the pioneering work of all these others. So I thank you!

REFERENCES

Alizadeh, A., Shahverdyan, G., & Etemadi A. The comparison of cognitive behavior therapy with psychopharmacological intervention for women with anxiety disorders *(GAD, SAD & OCD)*. *Psychology,* no. 3 (2012), 841–847. www.SciRP.org/journal/psych.

Amano, T., Unal, C. T., & Paré, D. Synaptic correlates of fear extinction in the amygdala. *Nature Neuroscience,* no. 13 (2010), 489–495.

Anderson, E., & Shivakumar, G. Effects of exercise and physical activity on anxiety. *Frontiers in Psychiatry,* no. 4 (2013), 1–4.

Armony, J. L., Servan-Schreiber, D., Cohen, J. D., & LeDoux, J. E. An anatomically constrained neural network model of fear conditioning. *Behavioral Neuroscience,* no. 109 (1995), 246–257.

Bachelor, A., & Horvath, A. (1999). The therapeutic relationship. In M. A. Hubble, B. L. Duncan, & S. D. Miller (Eds.), *The heart and soul of change: What works in therapy* (pp. 133–178). Washington, DC, US: American Psychological Association.

Barad, M. G., & Saxena, S. Neurobiology of extinction: A mechanism underlying behavior therapy for human anxiety disorders. *Primary Psychiatry*, no. 12 (2005), 45–51.

Billioti de Gage, Sophie, Moride, Yola, Ducruet, Thierry, Kurth, Tobias, Verdoux, Hélène, Tournier, Marie, Pariente, Antoine, & Begaud, Bernard (2014). Benzodiazapine use and risk of Alzheimer's disease: case-control study. *BMJ 2014; 349 doi: https:// doi.org/10.1136/bmj.g5205 (Published 09 September 2014)*

Black-Becker, Carolyn, Zayfert, Claudia, & Anderson, Emily. A survey of psychologists' attitudes towards and utilization of exposure therapy for PTSD. *Behaviour Research and Therapy.* Volume 42, Issue 3 March 2004, 277–292.

Bonchek, A. What's broken with cognitive behavior therapy treatment of obsessive-compulsive disorder and how to fix it. *American Journal of Psychotherapy*, no. 63 (2009), 69–86.

Bovend'Eerdt, Thamar J. H, Botell, Rachel E., Wade, Derick T. Writing SMART rehabilitation goals and achieving goal attainment scaling: A practical guide. Online research aarticle for Sage Journals: Volume: 23 issue: 4, 352–361.

Broocks, A., Meyer, T., Gleiter, C. H., Hillmer-Vogel, U., George, A., Bartmann, U., & Bandelow, B. Effect of aerobic exercise on behavioral and neuroendocrine responses to meta-chlorophenylpiperazine and to ipsapirone in untrained healthy subjects. *Psychopharmacology*, no. 155 (2001), 234–241.

Cain, C.K., Blouin, A. M., & Barad, M. Temporally massed CS presentations generate more fear extinction than spaced presentations. *Journal of Experimental Psychology: Animal Behavior Processes, no. 29 (2003),* 323–333.

Compton, R.J., Carp, J., Chaddock, L., Fineman, S. L., Quandt, L. C., & Ratliff, J. B. Trouble crossing the bridge: Altered interhemispheric communication of emotional images in anxiety. *Emotion*, no. 8 (2008), 684–692.

Covey, Stephen (1994). *7 habits of highly effective people: powerful lessons in personal change. US; DC Books.*

DeBoer L., Powers M., Utschig A., Otto M., & Smits J. Exploring exercise as an avenue for the treatment of anxiety disorders. *Expert Review of Neurotherapeutics,* no. 12 (2012), 1011–1022.

Desbordes, L.T., Negi, T.W.W., Pace, B.A., Wallace, C.L., Raison, C.L., Schwartz, E. L. Effects of mindful-attention and compassion meditation training on amygdala response to emotional stimuli in an ordinary, non-meditative state. *Frontiers in Human Neuroscience,* no. 6 (2012), Article 292, 1–15.

Dias, B., Banerjee, S., Goodman, J., & Ressler, K. Towards new approaches to disorders of fear and anxiety. *Current Opinion in Neurobiology,* no. 23 (2013), 346–352.

Dozois, D. J., Frewen, P. A., & Covin, R. Cognitive theories. In J. C. Thomas, D. L. Segal, & M. Hersen (eds.), *Comprehensive Handbook of Personality and Psychopathology, Vol. 1: Personality and Everyday Functioning,* (2006) pp. 173–191. Hoboken, NJ: Wiley.

Engels, A. S., Heller, W., Mohanty, A., Herrington, J. D., Banich, M. T., Webb, A. G., & Miller, G. A. Specificity of regional brain activity in anxiety types during emotion processing. *Psychophysiology,* no. 44 (2007), 352–363.

Fecteau, S., et al. Psychopathy and the mirror neuron system: preliminary findings from a non-psychiatric sample. *Psychiatry Res.* 160(2), (2008), 137–144.

Feinstein, J. S., Adolphs, R., Damasio, A., & Tranel, D. The human amygdala and the induction and experience of fear. *Current Biology,* no. 21 (2011) 34–38.

Froelinger, B. E., Garland, E. L., Modlin, L. A., & McClernon, F. J. Neurocognitive correlates of the effects of yoga meditation practice on emotion and cognition: A pilot study. *Frontiers in Integrative Neuroscience,* no. 6 (2012), 1–11.

Goldin, P. R., & Gross, J. J. Effects of mindfulness-based stress reduction (MBSR) on emotion regulation in social anxiety disorder. *Emotion,* no. 10 (2010), 83–91.

Gray, Shelly L., Anderson, Melissa L, Dublin, Sascha, et al;

(2015). Cumulative use of strong anticholinergics and incident dementia: a prospective cohort study. *JAMA In-
tern Med. 2015;175(3):401–407. doi:10.1001/jamaint-
ernmed.2014.7663*

Greenwood, B. N., Strong, P. V., Loughridge, A. B., Day, H. E.,
Clark, P. J., Mika, A., et al. (2012). 5-HT2C receptors in the
basolateral amygdala and dorsal striatum are a novel target
for the anxiolytic and antidepressant effects of exercise. *PLoS
ONE,* 7, e46118.

Grupe, D. W., & Nitschke, J. B. Uncertainty and anticipation in
anxiety: An integrated neurobiological and psychological perspective. *Nature Reviews in Neuroscience,* no. 14 (2013), 488–
501.

Hecht, D. The neural basis of optimism and Pessimism. *Experimental Neurobiology, no. 22 (2013),* 173–199.

Jantz, Gregory (2016). *Overcoming anxiety, worry, & fear.* Grand
Rapids, MI: Revell.

Jantz, Gregory (2009). *Healing the scars of emotional abuse.* Grand
Rapids, MI: Revell.

Jantz, Gregory (2013). *Turning your down into up.* Colorado
Springs, CO: Waterbrook.

Jerath, R., Barnes, V.A., Dillard-Wright, D., Jerath, S., & Hamil-
ton, B. Dynamic change of awareness during meditation techniques: neural and physiological correlates. *Frontiers in Human
Science,* no. 6 (2012), 1–4.

Johnsgard, K. W. (2004). Conquering depression and anxiety
through exercise. Amherst, N.Y.: Prometheus Books.

Kabat-Zinn, Jon. (2013) Full catastrophe living: Using the wisdom
of your body and mind to face stress, pain, and illness. New
York: Bantam Books.

Kirkwood, G., Rampes, H., Tuffrey, V., Richardson, J., & Pilkin-
gon, K. Yoga for anxiety: a systematic review of the research evidence. *British Journal of Sports Medicine,* Volume 39, Issue 12.

Kuhn, S., Kaufmann, C., Simon, D., Endrass, T., Gallinat, J., & Kathmann, N. Reduced
thickness of anterior cingulate cortex in obsessive-compuldisorder. *Cortex, 49* (2013), 2178–2185.

LeDoux, J. E. (1996). *The emotional brain: The mysterious underpinnings of emotional life.* New York. Simon & Schuster.

LeDoux, J. E. & Schiller, D. (2009). *The human amygdala: Insights from other animals.* In Whalen, P. J. & Phelps, E. A. (Eds.). *The human amygdala.* New York: Guilford Press.

Lewis, C. S. (1952). *Mere Christianity.* New York/London: Touchstone Books.

Li, Amber W. & Goldsmith, Carroll-Ann W. *The Effects of Yoga on Anxiety and Stress* Alternative Medicine Review Publisher, Date: March, 2012 Source Volume: 17 Source Issue: 1.

Linden, D.E. (2006). How psychotherapy changes the brain—the contribution of functional neuroimaging. *Molecular Psychiatry, 11*, 528–538.

Martin, D, J., Garske, J. P., & Davis, M. K. (2000). Relation of the therapeutic alliance with outcome and other variables: A meta-analytic review. *Journal of Consulting and Clinical Psychology, 68*, 438–450.

McRae, K., Gross, J. J., Weber, J., Robertson, E. R., Sokol-Hessner, P., Ray, R. D., Gabrieli, J. D., & Ochsner, K. N. (2012). The development of emotion regulation: An fMRI study of cognitive reappraisal in children, adolescents, and young adults. *Social Cognitive and Affective Neuroscience, 7*, 11–22.

Molendijk, M. L., Bus, B. A. A., Spinhoven, P., Penninx, B. W. J. H., Kenis, G., Prickaertz, J., Oude Voshaar, R. C., & Elzinga, B. M. (2011). Serum levels of brain-derived neurotrophic factor in major depressive disorder: State-trait issues, clinical features and pharmacological treatment. *Molecular Psychiatry, 6*, 1088–1095.

Muller, Wayne (2000). Sabbath: Finding rest, renewal, and delight in our busy lives. New York: Bantam Books

Muse, M. D., Moore, B. A., & Stahl, S. M. (2013). Benefits and challenges of integrated treatment. In S. M. Stahl & B. A. Moore (Eds.), *Anxiety disorders: A guide for integrating psychopharmacology and psychotherapy* (pp. 3–24). New York: Routledge.

Nader, K., Schafe, G. E. & LeDoux, J. E. (2000). Fear memories require protein synthesis in the amygdala for reconsolidation after retrieval. *Nature, 406,* 722–726.

Nolen-Hoeksema, S. (2000). The role of rumination in depressive disorders and mixed anxiety/depressive symptoms. *Journal of Abnormal Psychology, 109,* 504–11.

Oschner, K. N., Ray, R. R., Hughes, B., McRae, K., Cooper, J. C., Weber, J., Gabrieli, J. D.E., & Gross, J. J. (2009). Bottom-up and top-down processes in emotion generation. *Association for Psychological Science, 20,* 1322–331.

Otto, M. W., & Hofmann, S. G. (Eds.). (2010). *Avoiding treatment failures in the anxiety disorders.* New York: Springer.

Outhoff, K. (2010). The pharmacology of anxiolytics. *South African Family Practice, 52,* 99–105. doi:10.1080/20786204.2010.10873947.

Pascual-Leone, A., Amedi, A., Fregni, F., & Merabet, L. B. (2005). The plastic human brain cortex. *Annual Review of Neuroscience, 28,* 377–401.

Paul, Gina, Elam, Barb, & Verhulst, Steven J. *A Longitudinal Study of Students' Perceptions of Using Deep Breathing Meditation to Reduce Testing Stresses.* (pp 287–292) | Received 27 Nov 2006, Published online: 05 Dec 2007.

Peters, M. L., Flink, I. K., Boersma, K., & Linton, S. J. (2010). Manipulating optimism: Can imagining a best possible self be used to increase positive future expectancies? *The Journal of Positive Psychology, 5,* 204–211.

Phelps, E. A. (2009). The human amygdala and the control of fear. In Whalen, P. J. & Phelps, E. A. (Eds.). The human amygdala. New York: Guilford Press.

Phelps, E. A., Delgado, M. R., Nearing, K. I., & LeDoux, J. E. (2004). Extinction learning in humans: Role of the amygdala and vmPFC. *Neuron, 43*, 897–905.

Pittman, C. M. & Karle, E. M. (2015). Rewire Your Anxious Brain: How to Use the Neuroscience of Fear to End Anxiety, Panic, and Worry. Oakland, CA: New Harbinger.

Powers, Mark B., Emmelkamp, Paul M. G. *Virtual reality exposure therapy for anxiety disorders: A meta-analysis. Journal of Anxiety Disorders*. Volume 22, Issue 3 April 2008, 561–569.

Sander, D., Grafman, J., & Zalla, T. (2003). The human amygdala: An evolved system for relevance detection. *Reviews in the Neurosciences, 14*, 303–316.

Sharot, T. (2011). The optimism bias. *Current Biology, 21*, R942.

Sharot, T., Guitart-Masip, M., Korn, C. W., Chowdhury, R., & Dolan, R. J. (2012). How dopamine enhances an optimism bias in humans. *Current Biology, 22*, 1477–1481.

Siegel, Dan. (2009) Mindsight: The new science of personal transformation. New York: Random House.

Siegel, Dan. (2015) The developing mind, second edition: How relationships and the brain interact to shape who we are. New York: The Guilford Press.

Smits, J. A., Reese, H. E., Powers, M. B., & Otto, M. W. (2010). Combined cognitive behavioral and pharmacologic treatment strategies: Current status and future directions. In M. W. Otto, & S. G. Hofmann (Eds.), *Avoiding treatment failures in the anxiety disorders* (pp. 67–83) New York: Springer.

Stewart, Rebecca E., Chambless, Dianne L. Cognitive-behavioral therapy for adult anxiety disorders in clinical practice: A meta-analysis of effectiveness studies. *Journal of Consulting and Clinical Psychology*, Vol 77(4), Aug 2009, 595–606.

Sudak, D. M. Combining CBT and Medication: An Evidence-Based Approach. Hoboken, New Jersey: Wiley.

Taren, Adrienne A, Gianaros, Peter J., Greco, Carol M., et al. Mindfulness meditation training alters stress-related amygdala resting state functional connectivity: a randomized controlled trial. Social, Cognitive, and Affective Neuroscience, Vol. 10 (12), Dec 2015, 1758–1768.

Taylor, Steven, Thordarson, Dana S., Maxfield, Louise, Fedoroff, Ingrid C., Lovell, Karina, Ogrodniczuk, John. Comparative efficacy, speed, and adverse effects of three PTSD treatments: Exposure therapy, EMDR, and relaxation training. *Journal of Consulting and Clinical Psychology*, Vol 71(2), Apr 2003, 330–338.

van der Helm, E., Yao, J., Dutt, S., Rao, V., Salentin, J. M., & Walker, M. P. (2011). REM sleep depotentiates amygdala activity to previous emotional experiences. *Current Biology, 21*, 2029–2032.

Verduyn, P., Van Mechelen, I., & Tuerlinckx, F. (2011). The relation between event processing and the duration of emotional experience. *Emotion, 11*, 20–28.

Vreeland, B. (2007). Bridging the gap between mental and physical health: A multidisciplinary approach. *The Journal of Clinical Psychiatry, 68* (Suppl4), 26–33.

Walsh, R. & Shapiro, L. (2006). The meeting of meditative disciplines and Western psychology: A mutually enriching dialogue. *American Psychologist, 61*, 227–239.

Warm, J. S., Matthews, G., & Parasuraman, R. (2009). Cerebral hemodynamics and vigilance performance. *Military Psychology, 21*, 75–100.

Westra, H. A., Stewart, S. H., & Conrad, B. E. (2002). Naturalistic manner of benzodiazepine use and cognitive behavioral therapy outcome in panic disorder with agoraphobia. *Journal of Anxiety Disorders, 16*, 233–246.

Wilkinson, P. O. & Goodyer, I. M. (2008). The effects of cognitive-behaviour therapy on mood-related ruminative response style in depressed adolescents. *Child and Adolescent Psychiatry and Mental Health*, 2–13.

Wilson, R. (2009). *Don't panic: Taking control of anxiety attacks.* (3rd ed.). New York: Harper Perennial.

Wolitzky-Taylor, K. B., Horowitz, J. D., Powers, M. B., & Telch, M. J. (2008). Psychological approaches in the treatment of specific phobias: A meta-analysis. *Clinical Psychology Review, 28,* 1021–1037.

Würz, A., & Sungur, M. Z. (2009). Combining cognitive behavioural therapy and pharmacotherapy in the treatment of anxiety disorders: True gains or false hopes?. *Klinik Psikofarmakoloji Bülteni / Bulletin of Clinical Psychopharmacology, 19,* 436–446.

Yoo, S., Gujar, N., Hu, P., Jolesz, F. A., & Walker, M.P. (2007). The human emotional brain without sleep—a prefrontal amygdala disconnect. *Current Biology, 17,* 877–878.

Zeanah, Charles, H., Smyke, Anna T., Koga, Sebastian F. (2005). Attachment in institutionalized and community children in romania. *Child Development,* Vol. 76, Number 5, 1015–1028.

Zeidan, F., Martucci, K. T., Kraft, R. A., McHaffie, J. G., & Coghill, R. C. (2013). Neural correlates of mindfulness meditation-related anxiety relief. *Social Cognitive and Affective Neuroscience*, nst041.

Zurowski, B., Kordon, A., Weber-Fahr, W., Voderholzer, U., Kuelz, A. K., Freyer, T., Wahl, K., Buchel, C., & Hohagen, F. (2012). Relevance of orbitofrontal neurochemistry for the outcome of cognitive-behavioural therapy in patients with obsessive-compulsive disorder. *European Archives of Psychiatry and Clinical Neuroscience, 262,* 617–624.

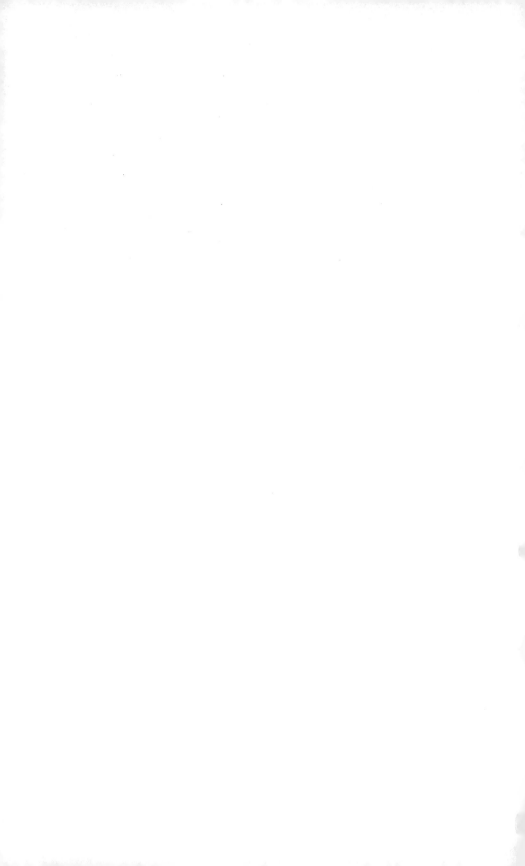

Order Information

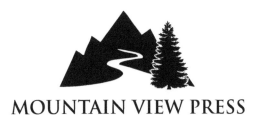

MOUNTAIN VIEW PRESS

To order additional copies of this book, please visit
www.redemption-press.com.
Also available on Amazon.com and BarnesandNoble.com
or by calling toll-free 1-844-2REDEEM.

Lightning Source UK Ltd.
Milton Keynes UK
UKHW042157230122
397588UK00003BA/35